The 101 Most Unusual Diseases and Disorders

THE 101 MOST UNUSUAL DISEASES AND DISORDERS

Evelyn B. Kelly

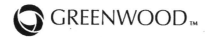

GREENWOOD™

An Imprint of ABC-CLIO, LLC

Santa Barbara, California • Denver, Colorado

Library of Congress Cataloging-in-Publication Data

Kelly, Evelyn B., author.
  The 101 most unusual diseases and disorders / Evelyn B. Kelly.
    pages cm
  Includes bibliographical references.
    ISBN 978-1-61069-675-3 (hardback) — ISBN 978-1-61069-676-0 (e-book) 1. Rare diseases. I. Title. II. Title: One hundred and one most unusual diseases and disorders.
  RC48.8.K45 2016
  616—dc23   2015023103

ISBN: 978-1-61069-675-3
EISBN: 978-1-61069-676-0

20 19 18 17 16   1 2 3 4 5

This book is also available on the World Wide Web as an eBook.
Visit www.abc-clio.com for details.

Greenwood
An Imprint of ABC-CLIO, LLC

ABC-CLIO, LLC
130 Cremona Drive, P.O. Box 1911
Santa Barbara, California 93116-1911

This book is printed on acid-free paper ∞

Manufactured in the United States of America

This book discusses treatments (including types of medication and mental health therapies), diagnostic tests for various symptoms and mental health disorders, and organizations. The author has made every effort to present accurate and up-to-date information. However, the information in this book is not intended to recommend or endorse particular treatments or organizations, or to substitute for the care or medical advice of a qualified health professional, or to be used to alter any medical therapy without a medical doctor's advice. Specific situations may require specific therapeutic approaches not included in this book. For those reasons, we recommend that readers follow the advice of qualified health care professionals directly involved in their care. Readers who suspect they may have specific medical problems should consult a physician about any suggestions made in this book.

I dedicate this book to my husband Charles,
my four children, and my four grandchildren.
They light up my life.

CONTENTS

ACKNOWLEDGMENTS

For a book such as this, one that has diverse diseases and disorders, I am indebted to many people, who have provided opportunities and training. I thank the staff at the University of Florida, who during my doctoral training, assisted me in learning about many of the disorders that affect children. I thank my many editors who have given me the opportunity to write over 400 articles. I especially appreciate ABC-CLIO/Greenwood Press for giving me the opportunity to present ideas to them for five other books. This one is my sixth book for ABC-CLIO, making a total of 17 books that I have written.

I am especially grateful to the American Medical Writers Association and the National Association of Science Writers for assisting me not only in writing, but in keeping up with scientific and medical advances.

Of course, no book would have been possible without the help and encouragement of my family. My husband, Charles L. Kelly, my four children, and my four grandchildren are my source of continued love and encouragement.

INTRODUCTION

How many diseases are there in the world? How many disorders can affect a human body? There are undoubtedly thousands, if not tens of thousands. Some diseases that were once common, such as smallpox, have all but disappeared from the Earth, and exist only in secure laboratory vials. Some are present only in the darkest recesses of the world's jungles or in remote areas, but with global travel and immigration, they are emerging into hospitals, with doctors admitting that they have never seen them before.

Diseases come in different sizes and with different effects. Some like influenza (the flu) are on the tips of people's tongues, especially during certain times of year. Some diseases, such as severe acute respiratory syndrome (SARS) or avian bird flu, get quick publicity and then disappear just as rapidly. Some disorders we hear a lot about because of constant advertising on television or radio. Such diseases as chronic obstructive pulmonary disease (COPD), osteoporosis, and mesothelioma were made household names by ads on television or in magazines.

These are not the diseases in this book. You have probably not heard of most of the 101 diseases featured here. You probably do not know anyone with uncombable hair syndrome or Pickwickian syndrome. Some of the disorders you may know by their characteristics or by other names. For example, you have probably heard of women who write to serial killers, but do not recognize the name hybristophilia.

I chose to compile the list of included diseases and disorders from various sources. As a medical writer, several of the disorders, especially those with genetic origins, I have written about before, but I have tried to choose some of the most unusual diseases, not just because they are unknown, but because they have an interesting or unusual component to them. Some of the diseases were suggested to me by other medical writers. I would never have known about burning tongue syndrome or Charles Bonnet syndrome without the help of these people. I hope you will find these conditions interesting, but please remember these diseases are real and affect real people, and should never be taken cavalierly.

PURPOSE

The purpose of this book is to inform and educate the reader about rare and unusual diseases. It is hoped that the reader will gain appreciation for the fact that these diseases are real and affect real people. Sometimes these diseases are called "orphan diseases," a name which has been changed to simply "rare diseases." While these conditions are rare, collectively there are many people who suffer from a rare condition.

STRUCTURE

The book is divided into five sections based on the causes behind these diseases and disorders. Each section includes an introduction that will give some background on the section in general. The introduction to each section will lay the foundation for understanding some of the terms used in the section.

The five sections covered include:

Unusual Genetic Disorders

Unusual Mental Health Disorders

Unusual Environmental Diseases and Disorders

Unusual Infectious Diseases

Unusual Diseases and Disorders with Other or Unexplained Origins

The resources list at the end of the volume will provide readers with information for further investigation.

Each entry in the book will include a fact box highlighting the most important facts about that condition. Entries follow the same general format, including a description of the condition and its causes, its signs and symptoms, how it is diagnosed, and how it is treated. Some entries also contain sidebars, which provided additional high interest information, such as personal case studies.

A WORD OF WARNING

Please note that information provided in this book may not be considered complete from a clinical perspective, as this book is intended for a lay audience who does not necessarily want or need to know all the medical minutiae related to a particular condition. And, in many cases, research into causes, diagnosis methods, and treatments for these conditions is ongoing. This book is not intended as a tool for medical diagnosis or treatment. If you have questions about specific symptoms or treatments, please consult with your health care professional.

PART I

UNUSUAL GENETIC DISORDERS

WHAT YOU SHOULD KNOW ABOUT GENETIC DISORDERS

Individual genetic diseases may be rare, but the number of people with genetic disorders is substantial. Of the approximately 7,000 genetic disorders, about 4,000 are caused by just one gene gone astray. Many of the disorders have no treatment. In the United States, in order to be considered a rare disease, a disease must affect fewer than 200,000 people; however, approximately 30 million people have different genetic disorders, emphasizing the point that a disease may be rare, but the number of people with rare diseases is substantial.

There are several reasons for choosing the genetic conditions featured in this section. Some of the diseases demonstrate some unusual features. For example, a child born with Cri-du-chat syndrome has an unusual cry, like that of a mewing kitten. Some disorders may be of historical significance. For example, King George III was thought to have porphyria, which caused fits of madness that impacted his ability to rule Great Britain. Other conditions are exceedingly rare, such as progeria, a disorder in which a child ages rapidly.

In order to better understand these conditions, some basic information about genetics is necessary.

GENETICS FACTS

It's All Done in the Cells. Each cell in the body contains a nucleus. Within the nucleus are 23 pairs of colored bodies, called chromosomes. One chromosome from each of the 23 pairs comes from each parent. On the chromosomes are the units of heredity called genes. The gene is a double-stranded segment of deoxyribonucleic acid (DNA), which contains the blueprint for making specific proteins. Four chemical bases are found on the twisted ladder of DNA: adenine, thymine, guanine, and cytosine. There are about 40,000 genes in the human body.

What Can Happen to Genes? Within the millions of chemical reactions, many things can happen. A genetic disorder can be caused by abnormalities in just one gene, or in the structure and number of the chromosomes. Genetic disorders are the result of mutations or changes in the genes. A mutation can occur in just one gene or in several genes that interact.

Chromosomes by the Numbers. Chromosomes are given numbers, according to their position in the cell. Somatic or body chromosomes are numbered 1 to 22. The last pair is made up of the sex chromosomes—X and Y. Chromosomes have a pinched area in the middle called a centromere. The "address" of the genes is given this way: those on the short arm (above the pinch or centromere) are located at "p" (for petite); those below the centromere are located at "q" (the letter following "p").

Inheritance Patterns. There are several ways a gene is transmitted to offspring:

- **Single gene dominant.** A dominant trait prevails in the presence of the recessive trait. Dominant disorders happen when an offspring receives a defective gene from either parent.
- **Single gene recessive.** The person must inherit two copies of the mutated gene. Most rare conditions are caused by recessive genes.
- **X-linked dominant.** Females have two X chromosomes; males have an X and Y chromosome. The X chromosome is large and carries a lot of information. If the trait for the disease is carried on the X chromosome, there may be nothing on the small Y chromosome to mask it. Hence, most X-linked genes occur in male offspring.
- **Y-linked disorders.** These conditions affect only men, as only men have a Y chromosome.
- **Multifactorial genes.** Several genes interact to cause disorders.

For Further Information

Gene Reviews. http://ncbi.nlm.nih.gov/books/NBK1116.

Genetic and Rare Diseases Information Center (GARD). http://rarediseases.info.nih .gov/GARD.

Kelly, Evelyn B. *Encyclopedia of Human Genetics and Diseases.* Santa Barbara: ABC-CLIO, 2013.

Lewis, Ricki. *Human Genetics: Concepts and Applications.* Tenth Edition. New York: McGraw Hill, 2012.

Marion, Robert. *Genetic Rounds: A Doctor's Encounters in the Field That Revolutionized Medicine.* New York: Kaplan Press, 2009.

Achondroplasia: Little People

- Also known as dwarfism
- Prevalence: 1 in 15,000 to 40,000 newborns
- Considered to apply to an adult with a height of under 52 inches for men; under 48 inches for women
- A genetic disorder of bone growth

Depictions of little people in Egyptian art reveal that throughout history, individuals who are small have fascinated others. The word "dwarf" appeared in a document dated 700 CE. Fairy tales such as Snow White and the Seven Dwarfs are familiar. Royal courts used dwarfs for entertainment. In the Prado Museum in Spain, Velasquez's famous painting shows the little princess surrounded by dwarfs who are entertaining the court. In the 1800s, traveling circuses found that a group of little people could attract interest. They called the little people "midgets," a term that is now considered improper and disrespectful. Achondroplasia is the scientific name, although most agree now that "Little People" is the preferred term. Achondroplasia is one of the oldest known congenital conditions.

WHAT IS ACHONDROPLASIA?

Achondroplasia is a type of genetic disorder that affects bone growth, and is the most common cause of short stature. The person has disproportionately short limbs. The gene that is responsible can be inherited as a dominant trait, but in about 80 percent of cases, the mutation in the gene is spontaneous with neither parent having a history of the condition.

The word "achondroplasia" comes from Greek root words: *a,* meaning "without," *chondro,* meaning "cartilage," and *plas,* meaning "form." However, the actual problem is not in the cartilage, but in the process of making or converting cartilage to bone. Cartilage is a hard, rubbery-like substance found in different parts of the body, especially the nose, joints, and ears. Cartilage is present at birth in some of the areas that will later transform into bone. As a child grows, the long bones in the arms and legs continue to grow. But with achondroplasia, the cartilage does not properly convert into bone, especially in the long bones of the arms and legs. This results in disproportionately short limbs and thus, abnormally short stature.

Scientists have located the gene that is responsible for achondroplasia. The gene is officially known as the "fibroblast growth factor receptor 3" gene or *FGFR3,* located on chromosome 4. This gene is known for making the proteins that regulate the growth rate in the long bones. However, if a mutation occurs in the gene, the receptor can become overactive and disturb the proper bone growth. The cartilage will not be converted to bone, and a shortage of bone cells occurs.

The gene is inherited in an autosomal dominant pattern. This means that if one of the parents has the gene, there is a 50/50 chance that the child will have the condition. Because it is carried on a somatic chromosome, both boys and girls can be affected. About 80 percent of children with achondroplasia are born to average-size people. As the normal gene mutates spontaneously, it is unlikely that the couple will have another child with the condition.

WHAT ARE THE SIGNS AND SYMPTOMS?

The most obvious symptoms are short, disproportionate arms and legs, causing reduced height. Other symptoms include a large head with prominent forehead, a flat or depressed area at the base of the nose, short fingers and toes, and hyperflexible ligaments in fingers. The condition is obvious at birth, when tests show that the child may have poor muscle tone. That delay in muscle tone continues throughout life; the child may have problems sitting, crawling, and walking.

Other health problems may affect the child. A hump on the back, called kyphosis, may develop and lead to curvature of the spine. He or she may get ear infections due to blockages of the Eustachian tubes. Problems with sleeping and breathing may also develop because of the compression on the chest. However, intelligence and cognitive abilities are normal, and most individuals with this condition have a normal lifespan.

HOW IS IT DIAGNOSED?

Prenatal ultrasound can determine if a child has achondroplasia. If both parents have the gene, a DNA test can be performed prenatally to see if the child has both mutated genes, which can lead to stillbirth.

WHAT IS THE TREATMENT?

No treatment exists for achondroplasia at present. Several researchers have experimented with growth hormones and surgery. Growth hormone therapy may be effective during the first year of life. However, currently it is quite expensive, ranging from about $10,000 to $25,000 per year. Another possibility is limb lengthening, which is quite painful and can cost as much as $100,000. Although their short stature may present certain difficulties, most with achondroplasia do not see a need to be "cured." Indeed, a strong support group called Little People of America (LPA) has worked to provide education and information to help little people reach their full potential. Many little people are successful in a variety of fields, including science, medicine, and acting.

For Further Information

Little People of America, Inc. http://www.lpaonline.org/.

Nicoletti, B., E. Ascani, V. A. McKusick, and S. C. Dryburgh, eds. *Human Achondroplasia: A Multidisciplinary Approach.* Basic Life Sciences (Book 48). New York: Springer, 1998.

ACHOO Syndrome: Inherited Sneezing

- Also known as photic sneeze reflex, photoptarmosis, sun sneezing, autosomal dominant compelling helioophthalmic outburst syndrome
- Sneezing in the presence of bright sunlight
- Affects 18–35 percent of population
- An inherited disorder

Sneezing is something that everyone experiences. Also called sternutation, sneezing is a sudden and uncontrolled quick burst of air out of the nose and mouth. It can have many causes, such as a cold, influenza (flu), sinus drainage, an allergy to pollens, dust, or molds, or a reaction to anything that gets into the nose. Sneezing is an attempt of the body to get rid of unwanted material and to clear the nasal passages. However, there is one type that has little to do with irritation in the nasal passages: that is called the photic sneeze, or sneezing in the presence of bright sunlight.

WHAT IS ACHOO SYNDROME?

ACHOO syndrome is a genetic disorder that causes sneezing when one is exposed to bright light. ACHOO is an acronym for **A**utosomal dominant **Co**mpelling **Helio-o**phthalmic **O**utburst. ACHOO is inherited in an autosomal mode of inheritance, which means that one parent with the disorder gives the offspring a 50-50 chance of inheriting it. Also, the pattern of the number of sneezes appears to be inherited. Other terms come from the Greek: *helio,* meaning "sun," and *opthalmos,* meaning "eye." In other words, sneezing is related to the naso-ocular (nose-eye) reflex when the eye encounters bright light.

The brain has twelve pairs of cranial nerves that pass through separate holes in the skull. The fifth cranial nerve, called the trigeminal nerve, is responsible for sneezing. Researchers speculate that a malformation in this nerve causes it to be overstimulated in bright light. This overstimulation causes the photic sneeze.

According to researchers, not a lot attention is given to this condition, and it is still poorly understood. Even those who have the condition may brush it off as an annoying inconvenience, with minor complaining. However, problems could arise if the person is operating vehicles or machinery that require precise movements, or in some other hazardous situation.

This condition appears to be an old one. In *Problems*, Book XXXIII, Aristotle (382–322 BCE), the Greek philosopher, wrote of a puzzling condition in which people begin sneezing when they go out into the sun. He mused that the heat of the sun caused the nose to react. Two thousand years later, Francis Bacon (1561–1626), an English statesman and philosopher, encouraged sneezers to close their eyes when going out into the sun. Using his inductive reasoning methods, he surmised that the sunlight made the eyes water and that seeped into the nose and irritated it. His inductive reasoning, however, has been shown to be incorrect.

In 1978, Dr. Roberta Pagon, a sneeze specialist at the University of Washington School of Medicine, when discussing sternutatory habits with a group of colleagues, found that of that group of 10, four members admitted they sneezed in bright sunlight. The number of sneezes ranged from three to 43. This group created the name ACHOO syndrome.

WHAT ARE THE SIGNS AND SYMPTOMS?

Most people with the condition may experience only one or two sneezes when they go out into the sunlight. But others may have uncontrollable sneezing when exposed to the bright sun. Some individuals have experienced 30 to 40 sneezes, one after the other. Sneezing is uncontrollable. The bouts may last as long as 24 hours. The sneeze appears to be in reaction to change in light intensity, and not due to a specific wavelength of light.

HOW IS IT DIAGNOSED?

There are no specific diagnostic tools, and diagnosis is based on patients' self-reporting of sneezing in the presence of bright light.

WHAT IS THE TREATMENT?

Antihistamines used by people who have seasonal allergies may be given. But mostly, people learn to use sunglasses, hats, or other protective coverings when going out into the sun.

For Further Information
Langer, N., G. Beeli, and L. Jancke. "When the Sun Prickles Your Nose: An EEG Study Identifying Neural Bases of Photic Sneezing." *PloS One*, 2010; 5(2): e9208. http://www.ncbi.nlm.nih.gov/pubmed/20169159.

Alkaptonuria: The Black Urine Disease

- Prevalence: 1:100,000 to 1:250,000 worldwide
- Rare genetic disorder in which the urine appears black or dark brown when exposed to air
- The body is not able to break down certain amino acids
- Clinical symptoms similar to those of rheumatoid arthritis

In an isolated monastery in the old Austrian Empire, the monk Gregor Mendel (1822–1884) worked diligently in his garden. He noted that the peas that he had planted had some unusual patterns. As he cross-pollinated, he took careful notes and developed a theory that some of the traits were dominant and some were recessive. When he presented his findings at a scientific meeting in the town of Brün in 1865, no one paid much attention. So his work went unnoticed for about 40 years. Around the turn of the 20th century, some new instruments revealed the internal workings of the cell. The work of Mendel was taken off the shelf, as doctors and scientists became interested.

One of the persons fascinated by the workings of the cell and the ideas of Mendelian inheritance was an English physician, Dr. Archibald Garrod (1857–1936). As he observed his patients, he noted that one family had a pattern that caused their urine to turn dark. He called the condition alkaptonuria, and dubbed it "an inborn error of metabolism." This was the first connection between the inheritance of a disorder and body chemistry.

WHAT IS ALKAPTONURIA?

Alkaptonuria is a rare inherited disease in which the body is not able to break down certain amino acids. This deficit causes a substance called homogentisic acid to build up in the cartilage of joints, skin, and other vital organs. This acid, which is in the bloodstream, is filtered through the kidneys, and leaves the body through the urine. When exposed to air, the urine turns brownish-black. The word "alkaptonuria" combines the name of the substance "alkapton," (which is homogentisic acid in oxidated form), with the Greek word *uria*, meaning "urine."

Archibald Garrod was a doctor at the Great Ormond Street Hospital in London. He had a three-month-old patient, Thomas P., whose mother brought him in because she was very worried about the deep reddish-brown stain on his diapers. When Garrod collected a sample of the urine, he found that it turned black when exposed to air. Garrod lived in an era of the heyday of the so-called "piss prophets." These men used urine not only to diagnose various ailments, but also to predict the future of the person. Although many of the prophets were charlatans, they actually had stumbled upon a useful diagnostic tool of testing urine—without knowing it.

When talking with the family, the doctor found that five other family members had the same problem. From these studies he coined the term "inborn error of metabolism," and presented his findings in 1902, linking the metabolic buildup of alkaptons to the symptoms of the condition. In 1908 at the prestigious Royal College of Physicians, he presented a lecture on alkaptonuria outlining his views of the mode of inheritance The proposal was remarkable for his time, because so little was known then about body chemistry and metabolism, and even less about genetics.

In 1958, a study was released in the *Journal of Biological Chemistry* that related the nature of the deficit in tyrosine metabolism to alkaptonuria. It was not until 1996 that the gene homogentisate oxidase (HGD) was discovered.

The cause of the disorder is related to mutations in the autosomal recessive HGD gene located on the long arm (q) of chromosome 3. Because this is a recessive condition, the person must inherit two mutant copies of the HGD gene, which means one mutant must come from each parent to develop the condition. Normally, the HGD gene programs for the enzyme homogentisate oxidase, which breaks down the amino acids phenylalanine and tyrosine. These two amino acids are essential for healthy metabolism. A mutation in the gene interferes with this process. As a result, an acid called homogentisic acid and its oxide, called alkapton, builds up in the blood. It is then excreted in large amounts through the urine. Over the years, the homogentisic acid begins to build up in other parts of the body. One of the first occurs in the cartilage, then in the heart valves, kidneys, and the prostate in men. More than 70 mutations causing a change in just one amino acid can lead to alkaptonuria, and all the complications of alkaptonuria.

Life expectancy of the person with alkaptonuria is normal; however, because of the effect upon body parts, lifestyle may be seriously impeded. The most promising studies have found that the herbicide nitisinone may reduce the acid buildup in plasma and urine; trials are being conducted in the United States and Europe. In addition, a person with the HGD gene may be a candidate for gene therapy.

WHAT ARE THE SIGNS AND SYMPTOMS?

One of the first clues of alkaptonuria is the presence of dark-colored urine on a diaper that turns black when left out in the air. However, many parents may not observe this sign. Generally, no symptoms that homogentisic acid is building up show up during childhood or even early adulthood. But ever so slowly, the pigment is depositing in the cartilage throughout the body. At about the age of 40, signs begin to appear. The condition may display the following symptoms:

- **Arthritis, especially of the spine.** The hips, knees, and joints between the vertebra show clinical symptoms resembling rheumatoid arthritis, although on X-ray, the appearance is more like osteoarthritis.

- **Darkening of the ear.** The cartilage of the ear may appear bluish. Also, the wax in the ear turns red or black when exposed to air.
- **Dark spots on the sclera** or the white of the eye, and also on the cornea.
- **Skin darkening in sun-exposed areas** and around the sweat glands; perspiration may appear brown.
- **Kidney stones and stones in the prostate in men.** The stones are common in more than percent of cases.
- **Heart problems.** The acid builds up on the heart valves, especially the mitral valve; coronary artery disease may develop.

HOW IS IT DIAGNOSED?

Blood plasma and urine tests can verify the presence; if ferric acid is added to urine, it will turn black.

WHAT IS THE TREATMENT?

At present, no treatment is effective once the symptoms appear. Some attempts have been made to reduce the accumulation. Large doses of ascorbic acid or vitamin C have been used but have not been effective in all cases. Some benefits have been reported from dietary restrictions for children but not for adults.

For Further Information

Alkaptonuria Society. http://www.akusociety.org/.

Ranganath, L. R., J. C. Jarvis, and J. A. Gallagher. (May 2013). "Recent advances in management of alkaptonuria." *J. Clin. Pathol., 66* (5): 367–73.

Amyotrophic Lateral Sclerosis (ALS): Lou Gehrig's Disease

- Diagnosed in about 5,000 people each year in the United States
- Affects motor neurons
- Small percentage traced to specific genes
- No cure currently exists, although extensive research being done

In August 2014, a new craze hit the media and went viral. It was called the ALS Ice Bucket Challenge. It proved to be a great idea to call attention to a disease that people have possibly heard of but know little about—amyotrophic lateral sclerosis

(ALS) or Lou Gehrig's disease. The idea was to fill a bucket with ice water, declare the person who nominated you for the challenge, and at the same time nominate three other persons to become candidates. The individual then dumped the ice water on themselves and donated $10 to the ALS Association for research to find a cure for ALS. Anyone who refused to have the ice water dumped on them had to donate $100. Celebrities such as Justin Bieber, Lady Gaga, Oprah, and even George Bush Jr. were part of the action. As of August 25, 2014, the ALS Association had raised $79.7 million for research, compared to only $2.5 million the year before.

WHAT IS AMYOTROPHIC LATERAL SCLEROSIS?

Amyotrophic lateral sclerosis is a disease that affects the motor neurons, which are nerve cells that control all voluntary movements. The disease is progressive, which means that it starts with a simple stiff joint or twitching muscle, then gets progressively worse over time. The motor cells eventually die. The disease itself is fatal, and at present, there is no cure.

Motor neurons are cells that have a unique design. They have three parts like other cells: dendrites, which branch out from the cell body and receive electrochemical signals from other neurons; the cell body, which holds genetic information; and the axon, which sends an impulse across a synapse or gap to the dendrite of the next motor neuron. Motor neurons are located in the brain, brain stem, and spinal cord. Those in the brain and brain stem are called upper motor neurons, and those in the spinal cord are called lower motor neurons. The upper neurons direct the lower ones to do all kinds of voluntary actions, like chewing or walking. The lower axons may be quite long. For example, the neuron that connects the spinal cord to the foot may be a yard long.

ALS affects both the upper and lower motor neurons. The motor neurons begin to degenerate, stop sending messages to the muscles to move, then eventually die. The muscles become weak and waste away, a condition known as atrophy.

Motor disorders have baffled doctors for many years. In 1824 Charles Bell (1774–1842), a Scottish physician and neurologist, was the first for discover the difference between sensory and motor nerves in the spinal cord. In 1850, Dr. August Waller (1816–1870), a British neurophysiologist, was the first person to describe shriveled fibers in a patient who had died with movement disorder. As the century progressed, Dr. Jean-Martin Charcot (1825–1893), a French doctor, made the connection between the autopsy and clinical findings. The condition is sometimes called by his name.

In the 1950s an outbreak of ALS occurred among the Chamorro people of Guam, which enabled researchers to make a genetic connection. Actually, no one yet has determined what makes a young and vibrant person begin to lose motor function and develop ALS. There are several types of ALS, at last count about 10, and some of these have variations. A breakthrough occurred in 1993 when scientists discovered mutations in the gene that produces the superoxide dismutase1, soluble gene or *SOD1* gene, which produces the SOD1 enzyme. Located on chromosome 21, this discovery indicated that at least certain types of ALS are hereditary. Scientists are studying other genes that may also be related to ALS. Estimates are that about 5-10 percent of cases are directly inherited from parents. Others are caused when sporadic mutations occur during the lifetime or may be the result of trauma, frequent drug use, or participation in contact sports.

WHAT ARE THE SIGNS AND SYMPTOMS?

In the beginning, the symptoms are very subtle and resemble those of several other disorders. The person may experience muscle twitching, called fasciculation, stiff muscles, cramps, or just weakness in an arm or leg. The individual may attribute the symptoms to various causes, from "sleeping wrong" on the arm or leg to overexertion. The person may then begin to speak though his nose or have slurred speech. When the complaints of general muscle weakness become more specific, a physician may then suspect ALS. The complaints may include problems involving skills using the hand, such as writing, buttoning a shirt, or putting a key in a lock. The individual may also describe problems with balance, tripping, and stumbling. However, regardless of where the condition begins, it will soon spread to other body parts, an indication of deterioration in both upper and lower motor neurons.

The rate of progression varies from person to person. The person will soon not be able to stand or walk. Difficulty in eating may turn to choking. The person will still have normal sensory and cognitive abilities, and can generally understand what is happening to him or her. In later stages, the person's breathing is affected, and he or she may have to use a respirator. Death can occur due to breathing issues.

HOW IS IT DIAGNOSED?

Diagnosis is not simple. It usually involves eliminating other conditions that resemble ALS. The list is long. Leukemia, HIV, polio, West Nile virus, and Lyme disease have some of the same symptoms as ALS. After testing blood and urine for all sorts of other diseases, a large number of other tests will be performed. Electromyography (EMG) is a special test that records the electrical activity in muscles; another test is a nerve conduction study (NCS) that measures electrical energy and how the nerve sends signals. These tests, along with magnetic resonance imaging (MRI), can determine whether the person has other types of motor neuron problems, and whether to consider ALS.

The average age of onset, with no family history, is 56; for those with a family history, the average age of onset may be 48. The person usually lives for about three years, though this can vary with the individual and type of ALS. Dr. Stephen Hawking, a famous physicist, has had ALS for over 50 years.

WHAT IS THE TREATMENT?

No treatment will cure ALS. Riluzole is the only FDA-approved drug for treatment, and it has only a modest effect on the symptoms. Most of the treatments are palliative and are designed to reduce fatigue, muscle cramps, and spasticity. Physical therapy and other exercises are recommended to help the person remain mobile as long as possible.

HOW A BASEBALL GREAT NAMED A DISEASE

Naming diseases and disorders is complicated. Many are simply known by their long scientific names, or they are named for the person who worked extensively with them, such as Alois Alzheimer and Alzheimer's disease. It is unusual for a disease to be named after a person.

During the depression years, following the stock market crash of 1929, baseball became a pastime for individuals. People went to the games to watch players who had great talent. One of these was a first baseman named Lou Gehrig (1903–1941). Gehrig not only had great skill as a first baseman, but played 2,130 consecutive games, and holds the record for the most career grand slam home runs.

During the 1943 season, he began to note that his performance was not up to par. He began fumbling the ball and slipping and falling when running bases. His wife Eleanor took him to the Mayo Clinic in Minnesota, where he was diagnosed with a condition with a very long name: amyotrophic lateral sclerosis. When he retired from baseball on July 4, 1939, he spoke before his admiring fans in Yankee Stadium and told of his appreciation for them, and how he felt that he was the luckiest man in the world. The disease with the long name became Lou Gehrig's disease.

Lou Gehrig died on June 2, 1941. He was 38.

For Further Information
Wakefield, Darcy. *I Remember Running: The Year I Got Everything I Ever Wanted—and ALS.* Boston: DeCapo Press, 1996.

Angelman Syndrome: The Happy Puppet

- Prevalence: about 1,000 cases in the United States
- An inherited disorder that affects the nervous system

- Rigid arm movements and facial expressions that resemble a puppet
- Caused by a mutation on chromosome 15

A child is born who smiles a lot, then cries as if she is in pain. She has some unusual movements, which one could say resemble the movement of a wooden puppet. The child does not meet developmental markers, and the parents know something is wrong. They may go from one doctor to another without answers. Eventually they are referred to a geneticist, who after some testing, tells the parents their daughter has Angelman syndrome (AS).

WHAT IS ANGELMAN SYNDROME?

Angelman syndrome is a rare genetic disorder in which a child laughs and appears happy, and moves like a wooden puppet on a string. The condition affects the brain and nervous system. Symptoms usually begin to develop when the child is about six months old, when the development of the condition takes a distinct course. The child may shriek like he or she is in pain, then suddenly begin smiling and laughing. Throughout an entire lifetime, he or she may never be able to speak more than 50 words.

Dr. Harry Angelman (1915–1996), who practiced medicine in England, had three mentally challenged patients with a number of similar symptoms. All of these children had a stiff gait and flailed their arms with a jerky motion. They laughed a lot, but then were prone to seizures. While on a vacation in Italy, he saw a painting in the Castelvecchio Museum in Verona called *A Boy with a Puppet*. The expression on the puppet's face was exactly like his patients', and their jerky, stiff motions were very similar to those of a puppet. In 1965, he published a report in the journal *Developmental Medicine and Child Neurology* titled "Puppet Children." Interest in the condition was almost forgotten until the 1980s, when the condition was recognized with his name: Angelman syndrome.

Chromosome 15 is the chromosome responsible for several disorders, including Prader-Willi syndrome and AS. In 1987, Ellen Magenis, a physician at the Oregon Health and Science University Hospital, was studying people with Prader-Willi (PW) syndrome and was amazed to find some individuals who had seizures and severe developmental delay. Children with PW do not usually have seizures, nor are they severely mentally retarded. In addition, when looking at the genetic profile, she found a mutation located on chromosome 15. In the brain, the AS gene is primarily expressed from the maternally inherited chromosome 15. In PW, the gene mutation also comes from the mother. However, this group of children had genetic mutations from the father instead of the mother. Dr. Magenis's discovery in genetics forged the way for the recognition of AS as a different type of disorder, and for the differences in genetic mechanisms of AS.

The Angelman gene is called UBE3A, and is located on chromosome 15 at band q 12. The following four different things can happen to this gene, which can result in AS:

- *Chromosome deletion.* In about 68 percent of cases, the chromosome derived from the mother is missing a huge piece of the area containing the UBE4A gene. This mutated gene affects brain development and is associated with a small head (microcephaly), language impairment, and motor difficulties.
- *UBE3A mutation.* In about 13 percent of cases, small changes occur in the gene from the mother, not the father. This could be a change of only one amino acid base. Children with this mutation function somewhat better than those with the deletion.
- *Imprinting center defect.* There are special genes, called the imprinting center, that control whether a gene is turned off or on. Abnormalities in this imprinting center cause the gene UBE3A to go awry in about 6 percent of cases.
- *Two copies of the father's UBE3A gene.* This condition, called paternal uniparental disomy or UPD, occurs when the mother's gene is absent, and two copies of the father's gene take over, causing AS in approximately 3 percent of cases. This group tends to have better cognitive function and less verbal impairment. Some children in this group may speak up to 50 or more words and make simple sentences.
- *Individuals with no known mechanisms.* About 10 percent of parents have normal genetic tests. The children are diagnosed with AS by their clinical behavior.

WHAT ARE THE SIGNS AND SYMPTOMS?

The symptoms of AS are similar to a number of other disorders, such as autism, cerebral palsy, and Prader Willi syndrome (PW), often leading to misdiagnosis and loss of precious treatment time. According to "Angelman Syndrome 2005: Updated Consensus for Diagnostic Criteria," presented in the *American Journal of Medical Genetics*, 2006, the following four symptoms of physical and mental development are consistent 100 percent of the time:

- The child has severe functional developmental delay, far behind children of that age. They will be slow to walk, learn new skills, and communicate.
- The child will have obvious movement and balance disorders. He may be extremely clumsy and unsteady, and lurch forward with stiff, jerky motions.
- The child shows inconsistent, often puzzling behavior. She may cry and cry, then break out in frequent laughter and smiling. The child is very active and very excitable. She flails her arms or flaps her hands often.
- The child cannot speak or can utter only a few words. He may develop a set of nonverbal skills that include grunting, pointing, or grabbing.

All the above symptoms are present in all cases. There are also some symptoms that are present in about 80 percent of cases. The following three conditions may be observed through medical testing:

- The head is very small. This condition is known as microcephaly (from two Greek words: *micro* meaning "small" and *cephal* meaning "head"). The small head measurement lags about two years behind normal growth.
- Seizures may begin at about age three. Sometimes the severity of the seizures decreases as the person gets older, but the seizures usually continue throughout adult life.
- Because this condition affects the brain, the child will have an abnormal electroencephalogram (EEG), which is a reading of the brain waves. The abnormal EEG may appear during the first two years, and can be present before the onset of other clinical symptoms, such as seizures.

Other associated problems can also occur but are only present in about 20 to 80 percent of cases. These can include a district facial appearance with a protruding tongue, wide mouth, protruding jaw, drooling, and movements of the mouth, such as chewing or sucking. The child may have troublesome sleep patterns and a fascination with unusual things such as water, crinkly paper, and plastics. As the child gets older, he may become obese and develop scoliosis.

HOW IS IT DIAGNOSED?

According to the Angelman Syndrome Organization, about 50 percent of individuals are originally misdiagnosed. This confusion may cause a delay in early intervention and personalized treatment. AS is diagnosed through a laboratory test called DNA methylation, which screens the DNA taken from blood. This type of test can detect about 85 percent of individuals with AS. Additional molecular genetics studies may be needed to determine the specific cause of the remaining 15 percent.

WHAT IS THE TREATMENT?

There is no cure for AS, but there are a number of interventions to tackle the social, educational, and cognitive challenges faced by children with AS. These children qualify for interventions at diagnosis, in a federal plan called an Individual and Family Service Plan (IFSP). This will put them in touch with people trained to deal with severe disabilities, specifically AS. A program called Applied Behavior Analysis (ABA) has been effective for many children with AS. People with AS are usually in good physical health, and some individuals have lived beyond 70 years. However, they must have complete care, often in an institutional setting.

SCIENTISTS USE NEUROIMAGING TO FIND OUT WHY CHILDREN WITH AS SMILE

One of the hallmarks of AS is the smiling and laughter of the child. However, that does not mean that they are finding some incident humorous, or that they are even happy.

Actually, scientists do not know why children with AS laugh and smile. They have sought the answer in a technique called neuroimaging, which takes scans of the brain. Using neuroimaging, researchers have found areas of the brain associated with laughter in normal individuals. There is a humor-processing pathway in the frontal part of the brain and a supplemental motor area of the brain that is involved in the actual aspects of laughing and smiling.

CT and MRI scans of children who have the deletion type of AS (the most common) brain do show there are some abnormalities in the humor-processing pathway. According to some theorists, the laughter in AS appears to be an expressive motor event, and not related to feeling. However, the children may experience a variety of emotions, though apparent happiness does predominate.

Most reactions of the child with AS to both physical and mental stimuli are accompanied by laughter. At the age of one to three months, they develop an early onset pattern of what appears to be social smiling, but this is probably more of a motor response. Later, they develop facial expressions of happiness that characterize the child's personality. One study found that 70 percent of the time, there were spontaneous bursts of laughter. Scientists agree that additional study needs to be done on both normal laughter and the laughter of the child with AS. This is truly one of the more interesting and unusual mysteries of science.

For Further Information

The Official Parent's Sourcebook on Angelman Syndrome: A Revised and Updated Directory for the Internet Age. Las Vegas, NV: ICON Health Publications, 2005.

Ankylosing Spondylitis: Bamboo Back

- Also known as: Bamboo back; Bekhterev's disease; Bekhterev's syndrome; Marie-Strumpell disease
- Prevalence: Between 0.1 and 0.2 percent of general population
- Condition that causes the vertebrae of the spine to fuse
- Probably a combination of genetic and environmental causes

Norman Cousins (1915–1990), a political journalist and teacher, was in the prime of his career when he began to have terrible back pain and stiffness. When it became progressively worse, he was diagnosed with an incurable illness called ankylosing spondylitis (AS), a disease he had never heard of. But Cousins was not one to give in easily. He found that when he laughed at comedy, the pain lessened. He began to explore the relationship of laughter and pain. Renting all sorts of comedies such as the old Marx brothers and Three Stooges films, he found that 10 minutes of hard laughing could give him four hours of pain relief. He wrote of his experiences in a book, *The Anatomy of an Illness as Perceived by a Patient* in which he presented the idea that laughter, hope, and happiness cured him of an illness that only one in 500 recover from.

The experience with ankylosing spondylitis led Cousins to investigate how the mind affects the nervous and immune systems, and to later found the Norman Cousins Center for Psychoneuroimmunology at UCLA. Currently, AS is part of a major initiative in research on the brain and nervous system.

WHAT IS ANKYLOSING SPONDYLITIS?

Ankylosing spondylitis is a form of arthritis that bends the spine. The joints of the vertebrae become fused, and the joints of the sacrum and pelvis become immovable. The individual has severe pain and moves stiffly. A structure similar to bamboo develops around the vertebrae. Bamboo is a plant that is seen in tropics and subtropics, which has a rigid outer covering that keeps the bamboo from moving. Bamboo spine develops when the outer fibers of the vertebrae develop a fibrous ring that affects the areas between the vertebrae, causing them to link with one another. The spine appears like a stalk of bamboo.

The term "ankylosing spondylitis" is from Greek roots: *anklyos* meaning "crooked"; *spondylos* meaning "vertebrae," and the suffix *itis,* meaning "inflammation of." The name portrays a bent spine that is bent, along with an inflammation of the vertebrae.

People can get AS at any age, but it typically begins in adolescence or young adulthood, with pain and stiffness in the back. It occurs more often in males and is most prevalent in the Northern European countries. However, cases in women may go underdiagnosed, because women have different symptoms than men. Although men may have problems with spine and back, women tend to have problems all over, including fingers, toes, and rib cage. An accompanying condition is a type of iritis, an inflammation of the iris of the eye.

AS has a long history. In Egypt, a 5000-year-old mummy was unearthed that had a bamboo-like spine. Galen of Pergamon (129–c. 210 CE), a prominent Roman physician, found a kind of rheumatoid arthritis in which the spine became very rigid, almost as if it was glued together. In 1858, David Tucker wrote a book about Leonard Trask (1805–1861) called *The Wonderful Invalid,* which told of an American who suffered from a contortion of the neck and spine. He had been thrown from a horse, and that accident was thought to have led to his spinal condition. Pictures from the book show Trask with his head completely bent over, as if he was always staring at the ground. Considered a medical oddity at the time, he later became the first documented case of AS.

Vladimir Bekhterev (1857–1927), a Russian neurologist who is well known for his study of reflexes, Adolph Strumpell (1853–1925), a German neurologist who discovered symptoms of AS, and Pierre Marie (1853–1940), a French physician, all studied and classified AS. Sometimes, AS is called by the names of these doctors.

Most scientists suspect that AS is genetic, and have noted several genes that could be involved. Over 90 percent of cases have a mutation in the gene known as *HLA-B27* located on chromosome 6. Several other genes related to the immune system are suspects also. However, having the gene does not mean that the disorder will develop.

WHAT ARE THE SIGNS AND SYMPTOMS?

The symptoms appear gradually. Usually, the first thing that one notices is a dull pain deep in the lower back or lumbar region. When the person is resting, pain seems the most severe, and exercise and movement may help. Sometimes, the condition may occur with arthritis with pain in other body parts, such as the hips and shoulders. This condition is part of a group of disorders called spondyloarthropathies, conditions that inflame the connective tissues; these diseases may also affect the heart, lungs, and other organs, such as prostate in men. Generalized fatigue is common.

As the condition develops, the fusion of the spine may be complete, and the person has the bent appearance. The individual may be so bent that his eyes can only look at the ground.

HOW IS IT DIAGNOSED?

There are no direct tests. Measuring the flexibility of the spine, MRI, and X-rays can show spinal changes. Tests for the genetic marker for *HLA-B27* may combine with these other tests to confirm diagnosis.

WHAT IS THE TREATMENT?

No treatment for the condition exists. The person must rely on medication, physical therapy, and surgery to relieve the symptoms. If the eyes, heart, lungs, colon, or kidneys are affected, those conditions must be treated.

For Further Information

Cousins, Norman. *Anatomy of an Illness: As Perceived by the Patient* (Twentieth Anniversary Edition). New York: W. W. Norton & Company, 2005.

Khan, Muhammad Asim, *Ankylosing Spondylitis: The Facts* (The Facts Series). New York: Oxford University Press, 2002.

Charcot-Marie-Tooth Disease: A Common Disease That Almost No One Knows About

- Affects the peripheral nerves, those outside the brain and spinal cord
- One of the most common genetic neurological disorders
- Affects about 350,000 in the United States of all races
- Caused by a combination of over 40 different genes

Bernadette Scarduzio was born with one of the most common diseases that almost no one knows about. As an energetic young woman, she was engaged in sports and many activities. However, within a few years she was completely dependent on a motor scooter to get around and needed assistance to perform the simple tasks of daily life. Her father, who also had a mild case of Charcot-Marie-Tooth (CMT), took care of her. Her grandfather and several of his nine brothers and sisters also had the condition. When her father died of a heart attack, she decided to become the "face of Charcot-Marie-Tooth," the most common disease that most people have never heard of. In 2012 she made a documentary movie about living with CMT, titled *Bernadette*.

CMT is an unusual genetic disorder, which is often seen in many members of a family.

WHAT IS CHARCOT-MARIE-TOOTH (CMT) DISEASE?

Charcot-Marie-Tooth disease is a condition in which the peripheral nerves are affected. The peripheral nerves are those outside the brain and spinal cord and provide direction to the muscles of the arms, legs, and feet. When a disorder affects the peripheral nerves, it is called a peripheral neuropathy. The word neuropathy comes from Greek roots: *neuro,* meaning "nerve," and *path* meaning "disease of." CMT is one of the most common inherited neurological disorders.

Three researchers have given the disease its name. Jean-Martin Charcot (1825–1893), a French neurologist who is known as the "Father of Neurology," published a paper in 1886 describing a disorder of the peripheral nervous system involving the muscles. Charcot's name is related to at least 15 disorders of the nervous system, including CMT. Charcot's pupil Pierre Marie (1853–1940) also contributed to the 1886 paper. That same year, a British neurologist Howard Henry Tooth (1856–1925) wrote about a type of muscle atrophy related to a neuropathy; he identified that it was not just a muscle problem. The disease then combined all three of the doctors' names.

This genetic disease is probably caused by a combination of 40 different genes. Mutations cause defects in neuronal proteins that affect nerve signals as they are conducted by the axons and the myelin sheath that wraps around them. The myelin sheath is essential for proper conduction of impulses. Most of the defects are traced to a section on the short arm of chromosome 17. CMT is divided into several demyelinating neuropathies, such as CMT1, CMT2, CMT3, and CMT4. Inheritance patterns range from certain genes that are autosomal dominant, recessive, and X-linked. Depending upon the type and subtype, CMT has a rather complicated system of inheritance. These subtypes have subtle differences, but all relate to the conduction of the myelin sheath and the peripheral nervous system.

WHAT ARE THE SIGNS AND SYMPTOMS?

CMT affects both the motor and sensory nerves, however, most of the nerves that stimulate movement are affected. The earliest symptoms appear to involve weakness in the foot. The individual will develop an extremely high arch and curled toes, called hammertoes. Hammertoes involve the contraction of muscles around the middle joint of the toes, making them lift up and appear like one is hammering. The person may develop foot drop, which is a weakness in the foot and lower leg that makes the person unable to hold the foot in a horizontal position. The lower leg muscles become weak, and the loss of muscle bulk causes the calves of the leg to look quite small, called an "inverted champagne bottle appearance." Numbness in the lower legs makes the person walk with a "slapping gait," which means the feet hit the floor hard when taking steps. This can lead to a loss of balance, stumbling, and falling. As the disease progresses, weakness in the lower limbs may necessitate the use of a wheelchair.

The disease becomes progressively worse. Later, similar symptoms may appear in the hands and arms. The hands may acquire a claw-like appearance. Muscle loss in the hands may make it impossible to write, fasten buttons, or even open doors.

Sensory cells then begin to be disturbed. The person experiences tingling, burning, or no feeling in the hands and feet. He or she may become insensitive to pain, heat, or cold. In addition, hearing, chewing, swallowing, and speaking may be affected.

HOW IS IT DIAGNOSED?

CMT has some specific symptoms, which can help with the diagnosis. The first clue is that the person has difficulty lifting the foot or making foot-drop movements. The person also may have loss of muscle control or atrophy, lack of stretch reflexes of the legs, and thickened nerve bundles under the skin of the legs. The physician may order nerve condition studies, biopsy of nerves, and DNA testing.

WHAT IS THE TREATMENT?

No known cure exists. The individual may be made more mobile with orthopedic surgery or braces and orthopedic shoes. Physical and occupational therapy may help maintain muscle strength.

For Further Information

Berger, P., P. Young, and U. Suter. (2002). Molecular cell biology of Charcot-Marie-Tooth disease. *Neurogenetics, 4* (1): 1–15.

Charcot-Marie-Tooth Association. http://www.cmtausa.org/.

Cri-du-Chat: A Cry Like a Cat's

- Also known as chromosome 5p deletion syndrome
- Occurs about 1 in 35,000 live births
- Characterized at birth by an unusual cry, sounding like that of a mewing cat
- Several physical and cognitive disabilities are part of the syndrome

In 1963, Dr. Jérôme Lejeune (1926–1994), a French physician, noted that several of his patients had an unusual cry when they were born. The cry sounded like that of a little mewing kitten. He called the condition Cri-du-chat, which means "cry of the cat" in French. As one who was interested in the emerging field of genetics, he analyzed the chromosomal makeup of the children, and found that the end of chromosome 5 was deleted. Dr. Lejeune was a pioneer in the discovery of several genetic disorders that result from chromosome aberrations. His other important discovery was that Down syndrome is the result of an extra chromosome 21.

WHAT IS CRI-DU-CHAT SYNDROME?

Cri-du-chat syndrome is a rare genetic condition in which a piece at the end of chromosome 5 is missing. Occurring in one in about 35,000 live births, it is the most frequent deletion syndrome in humans. A deletion in a chromosome means that part of one of the chromosomes is missing, and has been deleted. In this case, it is part of chromosome 5 located in the p area. A portion of each chromosome is pinched into two arms, called the centromere. The short arm is referred to as "p" and the long arm "q." For this reason the name 5p- syndrome (5p minus syndrome) is sometimes used. A number of physical and mental symptoms may also accompany this loss in chromosome 5.

This rare syndrome is caused by a problem with chromosome 5; an aberration that can occur in two ways. The chromosome may have a missing piece or changed piece. At the end of the chromosome is a segment called the telomere. This aberration is probably the result of a random occurrence during the formation of the egg or sperm. In other situations, something may happen to the chromosome that causes it to develop a ring, or to rearrange with another chromosome in some way. The area that is missing is on the short arm (p) of chromosome 5 at position 12.3. Regardless, all children with cri-du-chat are missing part of the chromosome that is essential for development, which results in the symptoms of the disorder.

WHAT ARE THE SIGNS AND SYMPTOMS?

The condition is readily identified at birth because of the unusual crying sound. This sound arises from a defect in the larynx or voice box and a problem in the nervous system. However, about one-third of the children will lose this cry by about age two. The child may also have characteristic looks: a round moon-shaped face with wide-set eyes, folds in the corner of the eyes, skin tags in front of the ears, and a small head circumference. The birth weight is usually low. A long list of other symptoms and signs may occur:

- Slow growth, along with weak muscle tone
- Body abnormalities, such as webbed or fused fingers and toes, heart defects, inguinal hernia, separated abdominal muscles, and hip dislocation
- Behavioral problems such as aggression, hitting, biting, tantrums, repetitive movements, and hyperactivity; many children are dual diagnosed with attention-deficit/hyperactivity disorder (ADHD)
- Cognitive delays that vary with the individual
- Speech and language delays
- Seizures

However, females reaching puberty may develop normally and conceive children. Males have been reported to have small testes, but sperm production is normal.

HOW IS IT DIAGNOSED?

The distinctive cry and physical problems at birth are the first clues. The children at birth have a distinct appearance and may possess specific appearances of their faces and body. Cri-du-chat can be affirmed by genetic test showing the deletion in chromosome 5.

WHAT IS THE TREATMENT?

Before 1980, children with cri-du-chat were immediately placed in an institution and given little hope. Research has revealed that with early intervention, these children can make remarkable progress. Although there is no specific treatment, there are ways that the doctor will suggest to manage the symptoms. Interventions with speech, physical, and occupational therapy should begin as soon as possible. For example, most children have difficulty with language. A speech therapist can teach them gestures and sign language.

For Further Information
Parker, P. M. *Cri-Du-Chat Syndrome: A Bibliography and Dictionary for Physicians, Patients, and Genome Researchers.* San Diego, CA: ICON Health Publications, 2007.

Ehlers-Danlos Syndrome: The Flexible, Rubber Body

- Prevalence: all types, 1 in 5,000 births
- An disorder characterized by loose skin and joints
- Abnormality in collagen that makes up the connective tissue causes painful symptoms and possible damage to internal organs
- Can be inherited

His friends at school were amazed that Joey N. could perform unusual feats with his body. He was the center of attention when he could lie on his stomach, put his legs over his head, and pick up a rock with his toes. He enjoyed these short-lived performances, but he soon found there was a downside to his feats. He had a condition called Ehlers-Danlos syndrome or EDS, in which he had to be extremely careful to avoid injury to his fragile skin, and had to be watched constantly for internal damages.

WHAT IS EHLERS-DANLOS SYNDROME?

Ehlers-Danlos syndrome (EDS) is a group of inherited disorders that affects collagen, the substance that provides strength to the connective tissue of skin, bones, blood vessels, and other organs. Without collagen, a person would be like a jellyfish, without form or structure. Defects in the connective collagen lead to symptoms associated with EDS, which vary from mildly loose joints to extremely life-threatening conditions.

The history of EDS is long and complex. Hippocrates first described the symptoms in 400 BCE. In the 19th century, several circus sideshows featured the Elastic Skin Man, the India Rubber Man, and Frog Boy, who could perform amazing feats with their bodies.

In the beginning of the 20th century, two physicians identified this condition. In 1901, Edvard Ehlers (1863–1937), a Danish dermatologist, recognized the condition as a distinct entity, and in 1908, Henri-Alexandre Danlos (1844–1912), a French dermatologist, suggested that skin extensibility and fragility were the cardinal features of the syndrome, which now bears the names of both doctors. In the 1960s, the genetic makeup was recognized. In the past, doctors had listed as many as 10 types of the disorder, but in 1997, they agreed upon a simpler classification that included six major types and a few very rare minor types.

The recognition of EDS is made more difficult because the symptoms may be present in other conditions; some people have even been suspected of being hypochondriacs because underlying pain and chronic fatigue is difficult to describe. Therefore, EDS is often misdiagnosed. Some people have even referred to it as "an invisible disability." Many physicians do not recognize the signs of this complex disease, and interest groups are trying to raise awareness.

Mutations in a number of genes cause EDS. Most of the genes provide instruction for making the proteins that assemble the different types of collagen. Other genes instruct for making proteins than interact with proteins that assemble collagen. Any mutation or change disrupts the structure, production, or processing of collagen and causes the defects that result in the symptoms. The major genes *COL3A1*, located on chromosome 2, *COL5A1* located on chromosome 9 are inherited in a dominant pattern. This means that one copy of the mutated gene is inherited from one affected parent. Rarer forms are inherited in an autosomal recessive pattern. Some forms may also occur, as new or spontaneous mutations occurring in people who have no family history of the disorder.

WHAT ARE THE SIGNS AND SYMPTOMS?

All types of EDS affect joints, and many affect the skin because of the defect in the collagen in the connective tissue. In addition to the general effect, the symptoms include back pain, easily damaged bruised and stretchy skin, joint dislocation and pain, vision problems, easy scarring, and poor wound healing. Most forms have hypermobility or joints with an unusually large range of motion. Infants with these type of joints often have weak muscle tone and experience delay in development of motor skills needed for crawling, standing, and walking. These loose joints are also prone to dislocation. Often in childhood, the child with EDS may appear to be abused, which can lead to embarrassed, frustrated parents.

One of the features of the person who has highly elastic skin is that it is very soft, fragile, and velvety to the touch. This type of skin bruises and scars easily. People with one of the classic types have wounds that split open with little bleeding, leaving "cigarette paper" scars.

The most serious types of EDS exhibit symptoms of the other types but also have serious life-threatening complications. For examples, blood vessels may rupture, leading to internal bleeding, stroke, and shock.

HOW IS IT DIAGNOSED?

The health care provider will perform an extensive evaluation, including family history. Tests include collagen typing based on a skin biopsy, collagen gene mutation, echocardiogram to determine if the heart has been affected, among other tests as needed.

WHAT IS THE TREATMENT?

Because this is a genetic disorder, no treatment for EDS now exists. Individual problems are noted and treated according to the symptoms. Physical therapy will be needed.

LIFE WITH STRETCHY SKIN

Sometimes people with EDS gain notoriety for their feats. On October 29, 1999, Garry Turner set a record for being able to stretch the skin on his abdomen 6.25 inches from his body. He was recorded in *The Guinness Book of Records* at their meeting in Los Angeles, when he also demonstrated how he could pull the skin on his neck up and completely over his jaw.

Turner described his skin as different from that of normal-skinned people. He said that if one looks at normal skin under a microscope, the outside layer of epithelial cells look like shingles on a roof, overlapping to form a nice protective barrier. But on Turner's skin, the cells look jagged, and do not fit together.

His nurse described him at birth as having loose skin. Growing up, he loved sports, but was always getting banged and bruised. Physicians diagnosed his condition when he was 13.

Turner now performs with the Circus of Horrors, based in Norwich, England. When asked about the pain, he said that he must use a small morphine patch to kill the pain beneath the stretchy skin. From the moment that he wakes up in the morning, he is in pain. However, he does enjoy performing in the Circus of Horrors, which is also the way he makes a living.

For Further Information

The Ehlers-Danlos National Foundation. http://www.ednf.org/.

Kahlman, Paul. *The Ehlers Danlos Patient's Sourcebook*. Printed by CreateSpace Independent Publishing, 2014.

Ellis-van Creveld Syndrome (EVC): Children with Short Limbs and Extra Digits

- Also known as chondroectodermal dysplasia or mesoectodermal dysplasia; formerly known as six-fingered dwarfism (now not acceptable)
- Prevalence: About 1 in 60,000 to 200,000 in general population
- Found more prominently among Old Order Amish
- A form of skeletal dysplasia, in which bones do not form properly

In 1744, Samuel King, his wife, and a small cohort of 200 German immigrants made their way to a beautiful area that is now Lancaster County, Pennsylvania. They were members of a group of dissenters called the Amish, who came seeking religious freedom. Into this area, one of the Kings carried a mutated gene that causes children to be born with several disorders. Over the years, the close group that became known as Old Order Amish intermarriedand passed the recessive gene to successive generations. The condition that occurs when there is a loss of genetic variation is called the "founder effect." A founder effect occurs when as close-knit group marry only within their own community and prevent new genetic variation from entering the population. Thus, children are likely to inherit recessive genes.

In the late 1930s, pediatricians Richard W. B. Ellis (1902–1966) of Edinburgh, Scotland, and Simon van Creveld (1895–1971) were riding together on a train to a conference in England. When they began to compare notes, they found they both had patients with the similar condition of extra fingers and short limbs. They agreed to do additional study on the condition, and in 1933 wrote a paper that appeared in a medical textbook. The condition became known as Elllis-van Creveld syndrome (EVC). About 20 years later in 1964, American geneticist Victor McCusick (1921-2008) studied a condition found in the Old Order Amish of Pennsylvania, and reported the genetic condition in this population, which was traced to the Kings. The condition Ellis-van Creveld syndrome occurs in about 5 of 1000 births with an estimated 13 percent of carriers in the Amish order.

WHAT IS ELLIS-VAN CREVELD SYNDROME?

Ellis-van Creveld syndrome is a genetic condition found in the Old Order Amish and in some of the populations off the Western coast of Australia. It is classified as a skeletal dysplasia disorder, meaning that the bones do not develop properly. EVC is seldom found outside these two populations, although it is possible.

Mutations in two autosomal recessive genes *EVC* and *EVC2* cause this syndrome. These two genes provide instructions for normal growth and development and work together to form heart, bones, kidneys, and lungs. When two recessive genes are inherited from parents, the child may have EVC, which produces dwarfism, heart defects, and other symptoms. The recessive mutation may be carried by parents who do not display the condition.

New studies have revealed that the basic cause may arise from a dysfunction of the molecular mechanism in the cilia structures, which are small hair-like structures that move molecules through the cells of the body. Studying the genetic pathways of EVC may shed light upon a large group of syndromes and diseases called ciliopathies.

WHAT ARE THE SIGNS AND SYMPTOMS?

At birth, the child has short limbs and an extremely narrow chest. Other symptoms are common: presence of extra fingers and toes, a condition known as polydactyly, congenital heart defects, deformed fingernails, cleft palate, and fused wrist bones. The child may be born with teeth or when the teeth do appear, they are shaped like cones. The disorder appears equally in males and females; intellectual ability is normal.

HOW IS IT DIAGNOSED?

Symptoms such as extra digits and short limbs are immediately noticeable. Genetic tests can reveal which mutation is in the genes.

WHAT IS THE TREATMENT?

Like most genetic disorders, there is no cure. However, surgery can correct the additional digits. Malfunctions of the heart, lungs, and kidneys can be addressed through medication or surgery.

For Further Information
Ruiz-Perez, V. L., S. E. Ide, T. M. Strom, et al. "Mutations in a new gene in Ellis–van Creveld syndrome and Weyers acrodental dysostosis." *Nat. Genet.* 24 (3): 283–6, 2000.

Epidermolysis Bullosa (EB): Severe Blistering

- Known also as "Butterfly Children" in the United States, "Cotton Wool Babies" in Australia, and "Crystal Skin Children" in South America

- Prevalence: 1 in 50,000 in the United States
- Skin blisters with just a slight touch
- Can be life-threatening if it affects other organs in addition to the skin

What would it be like to have an eternal sunburn in which the skin peels, or to always have a burn inside the mouth, as if you have just gulped a hot drink? That is what Jonny Kennedy, a resident of Great Britain, experienced during his 36 years. Rather than feeling sorry for himself, he decided to help others understand EB, and began working diligently to raise awareness about this condition. His last act before he died in 2003 was making the documentary *The Boy Whose Skin Fell Off* about his life and upcoming death. Jonny wanted people to know about epidermolysis bullosa (EB).

WHAT IS EPIDERMOLYSIS BULLOSA?

Epidermolysis bullosa is a rare genetic condition in which blisters form on the skin, then break and peel off. It is like always living with third degree burns. The term "epidermolysis" comes from the Greek roots *epi*, meaning "upon," *dermis*, meaning "skin," and *lysis*, meaning "breaking down." The term "bullosa" means "blister." The term describes the blisters that form on the skin, then break apart. The children are sometimes called Butterfly Children in the United States because the skin is fragile like a butterfly's wings. The butterfly is the symbol of the support group, the Dystrophic Epidermolysis Bullosa Research Association of America (DebRA). In other parts of the world, other names are used: "Cotton Wool Babies" in Australia, and "Crystal Skin Children" in South America.

Actually, the condition is divided into four types, and there are over 300 mutations of this condition. Following are the four types:

- **Dystrophic epidermolysis bullosa.** This type affects both skin and other organs. The word "dystrophic" relates to defects in body metabolism. The overall skin and some internal organs appear to be as delicate as a butterfly's wings.
- **Epidermolysis bullosa simplex.** This type appears to affects only the hands and feet.
- **Junctional epidermolysis bullosa.** Blisters occur at any site of friction and affect hands and feet. This type can appear in both children and adults.
- **Hemidesmosomal epidermolysis bullosa.** Very rare. EB is present at birth; however, it is difficult to distinguish between the types. Usually, the doctors just settle for the diagnosis of EB because all the symptoms need attention.

The human skin has two layers: the outer layer called the epidermis, which also has several layers), and the inner layer called the dermis. The outer epidermis is made up of overlapping layers of epithelial cells that are arranged like tiles on a roof. This layer is tough and protects the underlying structures, along with many other functions. Between the two layers there is a protein called collagen that anchors the two layers and holds them together to keep them from moving separately. People born with EB do not have this protein that holds the two areas together; the two layers may slip, slide, and rub over each other. If the skin is touched, rubbed, or hit in some way, blisters and sores will form in the area. The delicate areas are prone to infection, and over the years are at risk for skin cancers.

Several genes are correlated with EB. Mutations in the *COL7A* gene, officially known as "Collagen, type VII, alpha 1" cause the most common type of EB, dystrophic EB. In the normal body, collagens stabilize the skin and strengthen and support connective tissues such as bone, tendons, ligaments, as well as skin. The mutations in the genes disrupt the process of collagen formation. These mutations can be inherited either dominant or recessive pattern.

WHAT ARE THE SIGNS AND SYMPTOMS?

The following symptoms vary depending on the form of the condition:

- Blisters on the skin present at birth
- Blisters on skin when injured or with temperature change
- Blisters around mouth and throat that cause swallowing or feeding difficulties
- Hair or nail loss, along with dental problems
- Tiny white bumps called milia on the skin
- Cough or hoarse cry along with breathing problems

For every type blisters, are present at birth, and many others will form when the person is injured or the temperature changes. Blisters that form around the mouth and throat cause swallowing and feeding difficulties.

HOW IS IT DIAGNOSED?

The pediatrician first examining the child may suspect EB by just observing the unusual blisters. Several tests can confirm EB: Genetic testing, skin biopsy, special tests of skin samples under the microscope. Also tests may be run for the various complications such as anemia, bacterial infections, GI problems, and growth rate of the child.

WHAT IS THE TREATMENT?

No cure exists for any form of EB. The main goal is to keep blisters from forming and to avoid complications. Patients must receive careful care at home to prevent infection. Regular whirlpool therapy and antibiotic ointments are suggested to keep the sores under control. The caregiver must be on the lookout for complications, such as eye problems, muscular dystrophy, or periodontal disease. Some cutting edge procedures, such as protein therapy and gene therapy, along with the use of the drug interferon, are being studied.

For Further Information

Corradin, Silvia. *Living with Epidermolysis Bullosa*. Raleigh, NC: Lulu.com Publications, 2007.

Dystrophic Epidermolysis Bullosa Research Association (DebRA of America). www .debra.org.

Fatal Familial Insomnia: Sleeplessness That Kills

- Very rare; diagnosed in less than 40 families worldwide
- Caused by a prion that destroys brain tissue
- Fatal disease in which the person is unable to sleep
- Inherited in a dominant pattern

Around his fortieth birthday in 1991, Michael A. Corke, a music teacher from New Lenox, Illinois, began having trouble sleeping. Thinking it was stress related to his job, he paid little attention until it began to affect his mental acuity and memory. His health deteriorated. When he could not sleep at all, he went to the University of Chicago where he was diagnosed with depression and multiple sclerosis. Realizing he was not sleeping, the physicians induced a coma, but still his brain failed to shut down. He died in 1992, after his forty-second birthday. He had fatal familial insomnia (FFI) and had not slept for six months.

WHAT IS FATAL FAMILIAL INSOMNIA?

Fatal familial insomnia is a condition in which a person is unable to fall asleep, while his or her health deteriorates. He or she then dies within several months.

Sleep is the time when the body repairs and rests itself, making living bearable for each person. But a rare disease that is inherited and present in a few families keeps the individual from sleeping; this disease is fatal familial insomnia. This rare genetic condition affects a person in middle age, and is designated as a prion disease, similar to another prion disease known as mad cow disease.

FFI strikes the person in four stages, leading eventually to death. It is inherited in an autosomal dominant pattern, which means that offspring have a 50/50 chance of inheriting the gene. This disorder is different from most genetic problems in that the symptoms may not appear until the person is between 30 and 60 years of age, so that the individual unknowingly passes the mutated gene to his or her children before realizing the presence of the disease. In addition, the person knows the problem exists and that they are dying, unlike people with dementia, who are seldom aware of what is happening to them. The person is aware that there is no treatment or cure, and of impending death within the year.

Normal sleep enables the body to renew and refurbish itself. In regular sleep, four stages last varying amounts of time, then the cycles repeat. The stages of normal sleep are:

- Stage 1—The person is getting still and may be in a light dozing stage; the eyes are closed and the person is easily awakened. This stage may last five to 10 minutes. If awakened at this time, the person may say that he was not really asleep.
- Stage 2—The person is now in light sleep and has periods in which the muscles have tone, but then relax. Heart rate slows and temperature decreases, getting ready for deep sleep. This is a non-REM (Random Eye Movement) stage. The stage lasts about 20 minutes.
- Stage 3—This non-REM stage is where deep sleep is beginning; the person is entering a period of time when brain waves are slow. This stage might be called a transition between light and deep sleep.
- Stage 4—This stage is called delta sleep; the person may be disoriented if awakened. REM occurs in which eye movements are rapid. This eye movement is unusual, because all other muscles are paralyzed. Brain activity occurs in dreaming. It is in the deeper stages that the body is reviving and repairing itself. The body builds bone, muscles, and the immune system. This stage occurs about 90 minutes in the cycle.

In noting the importance of sleep to the body, one can see the problems encountered when a person does not sleep at all.

Fatal familial insomnia is caused by a prion. A prion is an infectious agent that is the result of a misfolded protein in the brain. In a person's genome, certain genes give instructions for making proteins, which carry out the many functions that they were designed for. Normally, the gene *PRNP* instructs for making of the prion protein PrP^C. The gene is located on the short arm (p) of chromosome 20. Something happens that causes a mutation or change in the gene. In this case, it is a single exchange of an amino acid that makes the protein. Consequently, the protein does not fold properly, and the misfolds affect the structure of the brain.

The structure of the brain affected in FFI is called the thalamus, an area deep in the brain. The thalamus is responsible for regulating many sensory and motor perceptions; it especially controls sleep. As prions slowly destroy the thalamus, the person's normal functioning of sleep is interrupted. Some electroencephalograph (EEG) readings show the person with FFI may have REM movements when awake; dreams are occurring when they are awake.

The discovery of prions is fairly recent. Dr. Stanley Prusiner in the 1980s described the misfolded proteins. There are several other diseases that also are caused by prions. In the 1990s, a disorder called bovine spongiform encephalopathy (BSU) or mad cow disease caused panic in Europe; some people responded by killing cattle. Another prion disease is Creutzfeldt-Jakob disease (CJD), which causes dementia symptoms. Kuru is a disease found among New Guinea natives who practice ritual cannibalism. North American deer and elk sometimes have a kind of prion that causes wasting disease.

WHAT ARE THE SIGNS AND SYMPTOMS?

The initial symptoms of FFI resemble other common diseases, such as dementia, end-stage alcoholism, and encephalitis. FFI was only discovered in the late 1970s by an Italian doctor. (See Sidebar: Case History: An Italian Family Battles Fatal Insomnia.) The onset may not seem a cause for concern at first; the person simply cannot sleep. Taking sleep aids do not help and in some cases may make the condition worse.

FFI manifests in four stages. It usually takes between seven to 18 months for FFI to run its course in the following stages:

1. The person begins to worry about not being able to sleep and becomes panicky and has hallucinations. This stage lasts about four months.
2. As the person is deprived of more sleep, the panic attacks and hallucinations become more noticeable to others. This stage lasts about five months.
3. Because the person is not getting the needed rest to repair and restore body functions, he or she begins to lose weight rapidly, and looks haggard and weary; mental functioning decreases. This stage lasts about four months.
4. The person becomes unresponsive. However, some cognitive functions are working, and he or she understands what is happening. This last stage of total sleeplessness lasts about six months and leads to death.

HOW IS IT DIAGNOSED?

Diagnosing the condition is very difficult, especially because there have been so few cases observed. The condition may be misdiagnosed as any number of other conditions, including multiple sclerosis.

WHAT IS THE TREATMENT?

There is no treatment or cure. The focus has shifted to helping the person improve their quality of life. Sleeping pills and barbiturates do not work, and may worsen the progress of the disease.

CASE HISTORY: AN ITALIAN FAMILY BATTLES FATAL INSOMNIA

Dr. Ignazio Roiter was a country doctor in Italy. His wife Elisabeta was a member of a very prominent family from Venice that traced its roots back to the 1600s. In the late 1970s, Dr. Roiter noticed that his wife's aunt never seemed to sleep, even with strong sleeping pills. In a few months her health deteriorated, and she eventually died one year after the beginning of the mysterious sleep condition. A year later in 1979, a second aunt developed the same condition. These women, who had been so alive and alert, became sleepless zombies. The medical experts of the day were puzzled too.

Elisabeta remembered her grandfather, who in 1944 was awake all the time—then died suddenly. The doctor and his wife began to think that this condition was possibly an inherited disease. Going back to the local church where many of her relatives were buried, the couple found such causes of death listed as "epilepsy," "fever," and "mental illness." From there he constructed a family tree, listing all those who had died under similar circumstances.

Off the coast of Venice is San Servolo, an island that housed one of the first mental institutions. Some of his wife's relatives had been sent there to live through their dementia. When he presented his findings to the medical profession, doctors did not agree that this was a new disease. His wife's Uncle Silvano came for a visit. He could not sleep, and his personality was changing rapidly. The uncle was taken to a sleep specialist in Bologna, who videotaped his decline. During the taping, he did not close his eyes, but appeared to have nightmares even when awake.

Uncle Silvano had willed his brain to science. After he died, it was removed and taken to a specialist in Cleveland. The specialist found that the hypothalamus was full of holes, like a sponge. Dr. Prusiner in California used this finding to propose that some diseases are caused by mutated proteins in the brain. The proteins take over the healthy ones and cause death. Prusiner won the Nobel Prize in Medicine in 1997 for his work with prions and their diseases. Recently, 27 other families around the world have been found to have FFI.

For Further Information

Guilleminault, Christian. *Fatal Familial Insomnia: Inherited Prion Diseases, Sleep, and the Thalamus.* New York: Raven Press, 1994.

Hemochromatosis: The Celtic Curse

- About 10 percent of people of Celtic origin are carriers of the gene; about 1 percent actually have the condition

- One of the most prevalent genetic conditions found in the United States
- Iron builds up in the system, and if untreated, can damage body organs
- Treatment includes periodically removing blood to prevent iron buildup

Susan T. always wondered why her grandfather was giving blood. She marveled that anyone would put themselves through that torture once a month. "It makes me feel better," he said. He also told her that if you have red hair and blue eyes, you may have what is called the Celtic Curse, an inherited disorder of people whose ancestors came from Ireland and Scotland. Later in life, Susan found out that her grandfather had a condition known as hemochromatosis and that she had it too—although it can affect people with any kind of hair and eye color.

WHAT IS HEMOCHROMATOSIS?

Hemochromatosis is a condition in which the body builds up the mineral iron. From the early days of the cartoon character Popeye, who got strength from eating spinach, the maxim that green leafy vegetables are good because they have iron has been promoted. But there is another side. People with hemochromatosis absorb too much iron from foods or other sources, causing a buildup in tissues that over the years can damage vital organs. The word "hemochromatosis" comes from the following Greek roots: *hemo*, meaning "blood," *chromo*, meaning "color," and *osis*, meaning "condition of." Thus, the blood has a strong color of red because there is an overload of iron.

Three kinds of hemochromatosis exist: primary, which is hereditary; secondary, found with other conditions; and neonatal, present at birth:

- **Primary hemochromatosis.** Most of the hereditary cases can be traced to the *HFE* gene, which was discovered in 1996. There are several mutations of the gene, most of which are recessive.
- **Secondary hemochromatosis.** If a patient is given many blood transfusions, he or she may develop iron overload. People with certain hereditary anemias, such as sickle cell disease, or older patients who have blood disorders may need blood transfusions. Other conditions, such as cirrhosis of the liver due to alcohol abuse, may also cause hemochromatosis.
- **Neonatal.** Present in newborns, this form is extremely rare, and occurs when the liver does not function properly.

In 1865, Armand Trousseu (1801–1867), a French physician, noted that the skin of some of his patients had a bronze color, which did not come from the sun. He suspected some connection to diabetes. In 1890, Friedrich Daniel von Recklinghausen (1833–1910) noted that excess iron in the blood could damage the pancreas and result in diabetes.

Although iron overload and hemochromatosis has been around for many years, it is still basically unsuspected because it is hard to identify early in life. People do not know about it, and many doctors fail to recognize it. If they do, it is not taken seriously. When Sandra Thomas found that her mother was diagnosed with hemochromatosis, she struggled to find out about the disease but could get little information. In 1998, she founded the American Hemochromatosis Society in memory of her mother, who died from organ failure because of the condition. The goal of the society is to help people understand the seriousness of this condition and what they can do to prevent serious complications.

People with Celtic backgrounds are most at risk for the hereditary hemochromatosis. The disease was assumed to be caused by a single gene, which was discovered in 1996. Most of the cases fall into this category. Mutations in the gene *HFE* are the cause. In normal individuals, *HFE* provides instructions for a protein located on the surface of cells, particularly in the liver, intestines, and the immune system. *HFE* controls the production of an important protein hepcidin, the regulator of how iron is used in the body. This hormone tells the body how much iron to extract from food and how much to release from storage sites in the body. When everything is working properly, about 10 percent of the iron is obtained from food and stored for use.

But what happens when one copy of the 20 *HFE* mutations is inherited? The person becomes one of the 10 percent who carry the gene, which can be passed to their offspring. If a person inherits two copies of the *HFE* gene—one from the father and the other from the mother, he or she will have hereditary hemochromatosis. Life may be very normal until about the age of 40. Symptoms may be very quiet until later in life, but the potential is still there. *HFE* is usually inherited in a recessive pattern and is located on the short arm of chromosome 6.

Secondary hemochromatosis has the same advanced symptoms as the primary type, but occurs in conjunction with other types of disorders, such as betathalassemia, sickle cell disease, excess intake of iron supplements, cirrhosis of the liver, porphyria cutanea tarda, or multiple frequent blood transfusions.

Causes of neonatal conditions of this disease are still unknown. Why the liver of the newborn or fetus shuts down is a mystery. Some current thinkers propose that genetic factors are not involved, and that the mother's immune system may produce antibodies that damage the liver of the child.

WHAT ARE THE SIGNS AND SYMPTOMS?

This condition is very difficult to diagnose because many of the symptoms are similar to those of other diseases. The person may feel tired and extremely weak. He or she may lose weight and have abdominal or joint pain. Many disorders have these symptoms. The condition may show earlier in men than in women, because women lose blood during menstruation. But as iron begins to build up in the body tissues, the person may develop several other symptoms. The woman may experience early menopause; both sexes may lose their sex drive. They may develop shortness of breath and generally not feel well. They may lose body hair. If they are given a liver enzyme test, they will show elevated factors. However, these symptoms are seen in many conditions.

Then, as if they have been hit by a Mack truck, the advanced symptoms appear. Hemochromatosis is now is full swing, with the following advanced signs:

- Liver problems, such as cirrhosis of the liver or even liver cancer, may develop.
- The person may develop diabetes with high blood sugar.
- Abdominal pain occurs that does not go away.
- The heartbeat is irregular; heart failure may occur.
- The joints and bones are painful; severe arthritis may develop as iron is deposited in the joints.
- The skin may take on a grayish or bronze color.

HOW IS IT DIAGNOSED?

Diagnosis first begins with taking a family history and looking at the patient's risk factors. One quick indicator is that the person has red hair and is of Irish or Scottish (Celtic) ancestry. Tests include looking at serum iron, a liver biopsy, an MRI, or a genetic test for *HFE*. If hemochromatosis is found early, serious problems can be avoided.

WHAT IS THE TREATMENT?

Up until the end of the 19th century, a procedure called bloodletting was a treatment for just about every ailment. With hemochromatosis, bloodletting is still the major treatment. It involves taking blood from the arm at regular intervals. This relieves the iron buildup and the overload that may attack vital organs. Advanced symptoms are treated according to the organ damage, although phlebotomy is also continued. The person's diet must also be controlled. They may eat only moderate amounts of iron-rich foods, such as red meat, spinach, or organ meats. They also must not use any supplements that contain iron or vitamin C, which increases iron production.

For Further Information
Gamson, Cheryl. *The Iron Disorders Institute Guide to Hemochromatosis*. Toronto: Cumberland House, 2009.

Hypertrichosis: Werewolf-Like Appearance

- Genetic condition related to X chromosome, and also chromosomes 8 and 17
- Causes extensive hair growth all over the body
- May also be acquired later in life
- Not to be confused with hirsutism, which is excessive growth of hair related to the male hormone testosterone

In the 19th century, several traveling circuses employed people who had unusual characteristics to be part of a "freak show." They had bands of very small people, whom they called "midgets," exceedingly heavy people, and people with excess hair. One of the people, Julia Pastrana (1834–1860) traveled throughout the United States as the "bearded lady." She had dark hair distributed equally throughout her body, including the palms of her hands. After her death it was confirmed that she had x-linked congenital hypertrichosis.

WHAT IS HYPERTRICHOSIS?

Hypertrichosis is an abnormal growth of hair on the body. It has sometimes been called the "werewolf syndrome," because the presence of hair made the person appear like an animal. The hair is not dependent upon the male hormone androgen and should not be confused with a condition called hirsutism, which is related to hormones. The word "hypertrichosis" comes from three Greek roots: *hyper,* meaning "more" or "over;" *trich,* meaning "hair;" and *osis,* meaning "condition of."

Hypertrichosis can be either congenital or acquired. The congenital type is present at birth. The acquired type appears after birth and could be the result of eating disorders, drugs, or cancers.

Hypertrichosis has been noted in history and may contribute to some of the myths about werewolves; people who were said to come out at night, especially on the full moon, as wolves. In 1648 Italian physician and naturalist Ulisse Aldrovandi (1522-1605) described the family of Petrus Gonsalvus (1556-?), who lived on the Canary Islands as the first recorded instance. Gonsalvus also had two daughters, a son, and a grandchild with hair growing on the face and body. Petrus was known as "the Wolfman of the Canary Islands." A painting of Petrus is in the Ambras Castle at Innsbruck, Austria. Sometimes, the condition is called Ambras syndrome because of the portrait in this collection.

Other individuals became circus oddities. These include Jo-Jo the Dog-faced Man, Lionel the Lion-faced Man, Wolfman, and the Bearded Woman. More recently, families with hypertrichosis have been found in Mexico, Burma, Thailand, and Nepal. All of the members of these families had hypertrichosis.

Several genes are involved as the cause. A dominant mutation on the X-chromosome may give the son a 50/50 chance of getting the disease. A female may get it only from the father. H. lanuginosa may be related to chromosome 8, but is thought to be a spontaneous mutation rather than inherited. The terminal type or werewolf syndrome is related to a genetic mutation on chromosome 17.

WHAT ARE THE SIGNS AND SYMPTOMS OF HYPERTRICHOSIS?

Several different types of congenital hypertrichosis exist. They are:

- **Hypertrichosis lanuginosa.** During embryonic development, the fetus is covered with lanugo hair, a very fine, soft, and unpigmented hair that protects it from the strong amniotic fluid. Children with hypertrichosis keep the lanugo hair after birth. The hair is usually silver or blonde.
- **Generalized hypertrichosis.** Men and women have lots of dark facial and upper body hair.
- **Terminal hypertrichosis.** This type includes dark, thick hair all over the body; the condition is also combined with severe gum disease. Probably this type is the one that is most connected with werewolf syndrome.
- **Circumscribed hypertrichosis.** Certain body parts may exhibit excess growth. An example is hairy elbows.
- **Localized hypertrichosis.** Hair is thick and dense, but only on certain parts of the body.

Acquired hypertrichosis occurs when the person is older. It may be the result of taking certain drugs, cancers, or eating disorders. Usually it is found on the face, upper lip, and chin.

HOW IS IT DIAGNOSED?

Diagnosis begins with observation, then continues with questions about what excess hair might be expected for age, sex, and ethnicity that are not related to the male hormone.

WHAT IS THE TREATMENT?

There is no cure for congenital hypertrichosis; however, if it is determined that the condition is acquired through drugs or improper diet, the main cause can possibly be eliminated by changes. Hair can be removed by certain external methods, ranging from shaving and depilatories to laser hair removal. Some medications are being tested that suppress testosterone.

For Further Information
Wendelin, D., D. Pope, and S. Mallory. "Hypertrichosis." *Journal of the American Academy of Dermatology* 48 (2): 161–179, 2003.

Ichthyosis: Skin That Looks Like Fish Scales

- A genetic disorder caused by 28 or more different genes
- Characterized by scaling, itching, severe dryness, and very thin skin
- Several types of ichthyosis ranging from a mild condition to a life-threatening type
- Prevalence: Mild type about 1 in 100,000; collodion type 1 in 100,000; harlequin type, very rare

The parents of Deb V., New York City, were told that their baby would not survive through the night. The doctor was shocked by her red, angry skin, but she did make it through the first two months in the hospital. Her childhood was pain-ridden. She had fevers, infections, difficulty managing heat, and soft bones developed from years of steroid prescriptions. But her parents were dedicated to her care, and she lived through those early days. Deb is now a professor in the graduate program in Child Life at Bank Street College of Education. Her mission in life is to work with and teach about medically needy children. Deb V. had a severe form of ichthyosis, known as congenital ichthyosiform erythroderma (CIE). This skin condition is basically unknown and quite rare; however, with good care, children can survive.

WHAT IS ICHTHYOSIS?

Ichthyosis is a family of about 28 skin disorders that are characterized by scaling, itching, severe dryness, and very thin skin; a few children with extreme types have other serious problems, such as holes for nostrils and ears. In addition, the buildup of skin and scales can result in body odor when bacteria or fungi grow between the skin flakes. Scales may cause wax buildup in the ears that leads to hearing difficulties.

The word "ichthyosis" comes from two Greek words: *ichthus*, meaning "fish" and *osis* meaning "condition of." All types have dry, thickened, and rough scaly skin appearing like the scales on a fish. The various types range in severity from a mild, common type called ichthyosis vulgaris to CIE, the condition that Deb V. had, to the deadly harlequin type of ichthyosis.

The skin, which is the largest organ in the body, has many functions. As the primary protector of the body, skin keeps things out that should not be there and protects the things that should be. It is a barrier to excessive loss of body fluids. The outermost layer, called the epidermis, provides the most protection, but it is this outer layer that people with ichthyosis experience as defective.

Ichthyosis interrupts the normal action of the skin in many ways. The scales can lead to scratching, which then results in openings in the skin. This article is focusing on three types of ichthyosis.

WHAT ARE THE SIGNS AND SYMPTOMS?

Ichthyosis vulgaris. This type is the most common, and accounts for about 95 percent of all cases of ichthyosis. This condition begins in childhood and is inherited as a dominant condition. That means that if only one parent has the dominant gene, the offspring has a 50/50 chance of getting the disorder. It appears as dry, scaly skin, especially on the legs, arms, and hands, and is more noticeable in winter. Other skin disorders may occur with it. *Ichthyosis vulgaris* can be bothersome and, like its name implies, unpleasant in appearance, but it does not affect health in other ways.

Autosomal Recessive Congenital Ichthyosis—Ichthyosiform Erythroderma (CIE) type. This type is carried by a recessive gene, which means that both parents, who do not have the symptoms, must carry the gene. The baby is born with a parchment-like covering called a collodion that cracks at birth and begins to peel within two to four weeks after birth. The eyelids and lips may turn out, revealing pink underneath. With this condition, the skin is always bright red, and the palms and soles of feet may be thickened. The peeled skin puts the baby at high risk for all kinds of infections.

Harlequin Ichthyosis. This very rare form is also the most serious. The word "harlequin" is from the old French, describing a court clown who dressed in clothes with colored diamond-shaped patterns. There is also a type of Great Dane that is called a harlequin because of similar patterns. But this condition is not humorous. In Charleston, South Carolina in 1750, Reverend Oliver Hart wrote that May Evans had a child whose skin was dry and appeared like the scales of a fish. The child had only two holes for eyes and ears and lived only 48 hours.

Harlequin ichthyosis is characterized by thick, diamond-shaped plates of keratin on the skin. Keratin is the substance present in hair and nails. The plates are separated by raw cracked areas. Other conditions may result from the tension between the plates: eyes appear as a bloody mass; the mouth is pulled to one side, the ears and nose are tiny holes, appendages are deformed, heat and moisture are lost through the cracks in the plates; and the child has difficulty breathing. This form of the condition is caused by the *ABCA12 gene* located on chromosome 2.

HOW IS IT DIAGNOSED?

The doctor can usually diagnose just by looking at the skin, but may order a skin biopsy. Genetic testing may also be performed.

WHAT IS THE TREATMENT?

Milder forms of the condition may be managed with heavy-duty moisturizers, especially creams and ointments that have lactic acid, salicylic acid, and urea, which help skin to shed normally.

Until recently, the harlequin type was always fatal, with afflicted persons usually dying within only a few days from either dehydration or systemic infections. In the 1980s, however, a new medication called isotretinoin was discovered. A child born in 1984 who was treated regularly has survived, and at this writing, is working as a sports coach.

For Further Information
Foundation for Ichthyosis and Related Skin Types (FIRST). www.firstskinfoundation.org.

Lesch-Nyhan Syndrome: Children Who Mutilate Themselves

- Prevalence: 1 in 350,000 in all populations
- An X-linked recessive condition
- Striking feature is self-mutilating behavior such as lip biting and head banging
- Build up of purines, a type of body chemical essential for making DNA and RNA

Michael Lesch (1939–2008) was a medical student at Johns Hopkins when he noted that two brothers, ages four and eight, had some unusual behaviors. In addition to having cognitive disabilities, the boys bit their fingers and arms and constantly banged their heads. Along with his mentor Bill Nyhan, who at this writing is a professor at the University of California, San Diego School of Medicine, he identified this as a genetic disorder, passed from the mother to the sons. They published their findings in the *American Journal of Medicine* in 1964. Three years later, J. Edwin Seegmiller (1920–2006) discovered the biochemical basis of the disorder. The generally recognized name for the disorder is Lesch-Nyhan syndrome (LNS). Although self-mutilation occurs in other syndromes, it is only one major characteristic of Lesch-Nyhan Syndrome.

WHAT IS LESCH-NYHAN SYNDROME?

Lesch-Nyhan syndrome is a genetic disorder that affects the way the body uses certain chemicals. The English physician Archibald Garrod, in the early 1900s, called such disorders "inborn errors of metabolism," and an error of metabolism has occurred in LNS. Normally, purines are chemicals that are part of tissues that make RNA and DNA, the elements of the genetic code. An enzyme called hypoxanthine-guanine phosphoribosyltransferase (HGPRT) controls the use of purines in the body. A genetic mutation causes this enzyme to not function properly and uric acid to build up in the body. This syndrome is rare, and the behaviors are quite unique.

LNS is passed down from mother to child as an X-linked recessive disorder; thus, it occurs mostly in boys. Mutations in the *HPRT1* gene cause the syndrome. Normally, *HPRT1* instructs for the making of the enzyme HGPRT, which enables cells to recycle purines for the manufacture of DNA and RNA. This system is very efficient, and the smallest disruption can cause problems. More than 200 mutations of the *HPRT*1 gene exist. Most of the mutations involve only one exchange of a building block or nucleotide. The small exchange can cause shut down or malfunction. *HPRT*1 is located on the long arm (p) of the X chromosome.

WHAT ARE THE SIGNS AND SYMPTOMS?

When the enzyme HGPRT does not work properly, uric acid builds up in the system, causing a number of physical, cognitive, and behavioral symptoms. The first indication of the disease is the orange-colored, sand-like crystals of uric acid on the baby's diaper. Uric acid builds up in the body and affects the joints, causing a type of arthritis called gout. Kidney and bladder stones also develop.

Uric acid affects the nervous system. The most common symptoms that become noticeable, at about three to six months, are poor muscle tone and developmental delay. The child is late sitting up and almost never learns to walk, crawl, or speak. There may be other abnormal movements, such as arching the back, writhing, and spasticity. By age of two or three, behavioral disturbances emerge. He may make involuntary faces, called grimacing. He begins to injure himself. First, it appears as biting the lips or fingers. Later, it may turn into head banging. About 85 percent of children with the condition display these compulsive behaviors and as they grow older, display aggressiveness, vomiting, or spitting.

HOW IS IT DIAGNOSED?

The doctor will ask if there is a family history of this disorder. He will also perform an exam that will show over-exaggerated reflexes or spasticity. Blood and urine will show high uric acid levels. Genetic testing verifies the diagnosis.

WHAT IS THE TREATMENT?

Most of the treatment procedures target the symptoms. Gout can be treated with allopurinol to control excessive uric acid. If kidney or bladder stones develop, they can be treated with lithotripsy. No specific treatments exist for the neurological symptoms, although some behavioral interventions may help.

The prognosis for LNS is likely to be poor. Death may occur in the first or second decade, though with careful medical and psychological care, some individuals have lived into their twenties and beyond.

For Further Information
The Lesch-Nyhan Disease International Study Group. www.lesch-nyhan.org.

Porphyria: A Royal Condition

- Prevalence 1 in 25,000 in the United States
- Caused by a mutation in one of eight different genes
- Disorder of the mechanism that makes heme, the main ingredient of hemoglobin
- Can result in many physical and mental disturbances

George III of the Royal House of Hanover was king of Great Britain during the American Revolutionary War. He was known for his fits of madness, abdominal pain, reddish urine, and rashes; physicians treated him with the best-known treatment at the time: arsenic. Several members of the royal family were suspected of having a similar disorder. It has been proposed that King George had a condition known as porphyria, whose name fits the symbol of royalty, the color purple. The name comes from an ancient Greek word *porphura*, meaning "purple." The condition, which can manifest as eight types, not only has an important place in history, but is still present today as quite a challenging condition.

WHAT IS PORPHYRIA?

The porphyrias are a group of rare, genetic disorders in which the enzymes that produce porphyrins or heme do not work properly. The Greek word *heme* means "blood" and refers to the substance that gives blood its red color. Heme is the basic ingredient of the iron-containing proteins that make up hemoglobin, and is an important molecule for every organ in the body, including the blood, bone marrow, and liver. When these enzymes that make heme malfunction, the person may have neurological or skin problems, or both.

Although there are several types of porphyrins, they are usually classified into two groups: acute, which primarily affect the nervous and gastrointestinal systems, and cutaneous, which affects the skin, causing blisters, scarring, and infection. There are about eight types; six of these are extremely rare. However, all types have the same thing in common: the malfunction of the enzyme that produces heme.

Porphyria has an important history. The Greeks borrowed the word from the Phoenicians who made a purple dye from a special mollusk. The Phoenicians began the practice of robing the royal heir in purple and draping the king's palatial room with beautiful purple cloth. The term "born to the purple" was later used to describe one who is heir to the throne. The ancient people had no idea that the term would, some day, be used to describe a serious disorder that would be passed down through royal blood lines.

Hippocrates (c. 460–377 BCE), the famous Greek physician, was the first to recognize porphyria as a disease, which he believed came from the blood or liver. He noted that the urine of these patients became purple or red when exposed to light. The disorder has not escaped folklore. Several historians have theorized that the origins of vampires and werewolves legends were related to the condition porphyria. Individuals with cutaneous porphyria can become disfigured and grow excessive face and body hair. Because these people did not want to come out into the sun during the day, they were thought to be werewolves or even vampires who inhabited the night.

During the Middle Ages, medical "practitioners" called "piss prophets" used a patient's urine and feces as an important tool for diagnosis. However, in 1871, the new field of biochemistry was just developing, and German biochemist Felix Hoppe-Seyler (1825–1895) discovered the role of pigments in the blood. In 1889 Dutch physician Barend Jospeh Stokvis (1834–1902) described the pigments in the urine, and called them porphyrins.

Regardless of the type, all the disorders have one thing in common: the problem with the heme-building machinery. Heme, the major element in hemoglobin in the blood, is the main transporter of oxygen to the cells and the collector of carbon dioxide to be excreted. Heme is made in the body in an assembly line in eight steps. Each of these steps is controlled by a different enzyme. If there is a failure in any one of the steps, the whole machinery can break down, and incomplete products from the earlier steps can flood into the blood stream and build up to toxic levels. The porphyrins first accumulate in the skin and other organs, then are excreted in the urine and feces. Depending on where the breakdown was in the process, different symptoms and types may occur.

Mutations in one of eight different genes are related to porphyria. And although genetic mutations usually cause the accumulation of porphyrins, toxins such as alcohol or environmental contaminants can cause the disease. Probably the most unusual example of environmental contamination occurred in the 1950s in Turkey, when 4,000 people developed porphyria from ingesting wheat seeds that had been sprayed with the fungus-killing chemical hexachlorobenzene. In addition, other things may trigger an acute attack. A number of drugs, including sulfonamides, barbiturates, and some anesthetics, can also evoke an attack.

WHAT ARE THE SIGNS AND SYMPTOMS?

There are eight types of porphyria, which are divided into two basic groups: acute and cutaneous.

Acute porphyria. Following are the symptoms of this type, which affects the nervous system:

- Seizure and mental disturbances including hallucinations, depression, anxiety, and paranoia
- Gastrointestinal disturbances including abdominal pain, vomiting, constipation
- Acute neuropathy (a lack of feeling in the extremities) and muscle weakness
- Cardiac arrhythmias, especially high heart rate
- Severe general pain

Most porphyrias are genetic, but some patients who have certain other diseases, such as liver disease, may develop porphyria along with other signs, such as jaundice.

Cutaneous porphyria. Following are the symptoms of this type:

- Primarily affects the skin, causing blisters, itching, and swelling
- Gums deteriorate
- Increased hair growth on exposed areas, such as the forehead
- Urine turns purplish-red when exposed to sunlight

People with this type may not have abdominal pain, which can distinguish it from other types. This type may be more prevalent than once thought, because the condition is often misdiagnosed.

HOW IS IT DIAGNOSED?

If the disorder is suspected, the most obvious is biochemical analysis of urine, which will contain porphobilinogen (PGB) in every one of the types. Genetic tests are also performed.

WHAT IS THE TREATMENT?

Porphyria may be difficult to treat and manage. People will usually go to the doctor for many of the symptoms, such as gastrointestinal disturbances or skin disorders. Because mental and emotional distress may come and go, the possibility of misdiagnosis is always present. The acute type may have sudden severe symptoms. When it is definitely diagnosed, the person may need blood or heme transfusions or other treatments. Sometimes, a high carbohydrate diet is recommended. It is also recommended that the individual wear an identification bracelet in case of an accident or reaction to certain triggers.

VINCENT VAN GOGH AND ACUTE INTERMITTENT PORPHYRIA

In the tiny village of Auvers-sur-Oise, France, Vincent van Gogh, the talented French painter, lived and then died from a self-inflicted gunshot wound. It is a short walk up the hill to the cemetery, and the tombstone that reads "Ici Repose Vincent van Gogh 1853–1890." He was a prolific painter who once created 80 paintings in 70 days, but only sold one painting during his short lifetime. Some art historians believe that he had acute intermittent porphyria.

His lifelong illnesses have all the hallmarks of the disease. From his prolific letters to friends and family, he often complained of gastrointestinal problems and neurological disturbances. He had at least one bout of constipation that required medical intervention, and psychotic incidences that involved both auditory and visual hallucinations and seizures. Once, in a period of confusion, he cut off his own ear and gave it to a prostitute. His habit of drinking absinthe, a type of poisonous alcohol, might have been a trigger for porphyria. He was also known to eat lead-laden paint chips, which some have surmised resulted in his preference for the color yellow and bright colors. In addition, he complained of intermittent eye problems. The acute porphyria theory is supported by the fact that there were cases of mental illness in his family. Three of six children in his immediate family showed similar signs of acute intermittent porphyria.

For Further Information

American Porphyria Foundation. www.porphyriafoundation.com.

Deats-O'Reilly, Diana. *Porphyria: The Unknown Disease.* Grand Forks, ND: Porphyrin Press, 1998.

Prader-Willi Syndrome: The Padlocked Refrigerator

- Prevalence: 12,000 to 15,000 people
- Most common genetic condition that causes obesity
- Caused by a spontaneous genetic mutation located on chromosome 15
- Early signs and symptoms range from poor muscle tone to behavioral problems

Jessie's family knows that he has several problems. He is always hungry. At the end of a large meal, he will say to his mom, "I am still really hungry." He is 10 now and weighs 350 pounds. He has been diagnosed with Prader-Willi syndrome (PWS), a condition caused by a flaw in chromosome 15. His days are filled with hunger. The kitchen cabinets are on full lockdown; the refrigerator is padlocked with a special lock purchased from the Prader-Willi Syndrome Association. The family even has to lock up the dog food. Jessie has to be watched every minute, because he does not chew his food; he swallows it whole, and is likely to choke.

WHAT IS PRADER-WILLI SYNDROME?

Prader-Willi Syndrome (PWS) is a complex genetic disorder that affects behavior, growth, appetite, and cognitive ability. Some of the indications may show up during the prenatal period, and then each stage of development has different manifestations. One of the main attributes is the desire for constant eating. It is not unusual for the family to have to padlock cabinets and refrigerators. Overeating leads to obesity, which will lead to serious, life-threatening disorders. Also, the person may exhibit cognitive disorders, which can range from mild to severe.

Andrea Prader (1919–2001) first described the condition in 1956. Another Swiss physician, Heinrich Willi (1900–1971), also studied the condition. The name Prader-Willi was given in honor of these two physicians. Yet, physicians had no idea why people had this unusual collection of symptoms and features. In 1981, Dr. David Ledbetter found that in about 70 percent of cases, a large segment of genetic information on chromosome 15 is missing. The missing parts of the chromosome appear to disrupt the normal functioning of the hypothalamus, which controls appetite.

For unknown reasons, an error at the time of conception affects genes in a certain area of chromosome 15. This causes a flaw in the hypothalamus, the part of the brain that controls hunger. The flaw makes the person always hungry, with a continuous urge to eat that he cannot control. In addition, because of the poor muscle tone, the person needs less food and fewer calories.

There are three genetic forms of PWS:

- Paternal deletion, which causes about 70 percent of cases. A deletion simply means that part of the chromosome inherited from the father is missing.
- Maternal uniparental disomy, which occurs in about 25 percent of cases. In this form, the baby gets both copies from one parent. The word "maternal" means mother; "uniparental" means one parent; "disomy" means two chromosome bodies. It is thought that the mother's eggs had three copies and then lost one of the chromosomes. With this type, the person may have additional genetic disorders.
- Imprinting, which occurs in less than 5 percent of cases. In very rare instances, the genes on chromosome 15 are present, but they simply do not work. A small section of the chromosome controls imprinting, and in this case, it is not working. The defect may be in the father's genes or it can appear suddenly with no explanation.

WHAT ARE THE SIGNS AND SYMPTOMS?

The first signs of PWS may begin in the uterus and at birth. The mother may experience reduced fetal movement and frequent abnormal fetal position. The mother may also have excessive amniotic fluid, a condition known as polyhydramnios. The birth may be breech, requiring a caesarean section. When the child is born, he or she may have a variety of symptoms, such as poor eye coordination and muscle tone. One of the major issues is the failure to thrive. The child's cry is weak, and he or she may have difficulty waking up. One other initial sign is a thin upper lip and almond-shaped eyes, with a down-turned mouth.

Childhood brings other problems. The person may sleep excessively and experience delayed development, especially intellectual and speech delay. Overeating or hyperphagia begins around the age of two and continues throughout adulthood. The child does not chew his or her food, but appears to swallow it whole. The child is usually short, and may display scoliosis at this time. Behavioral problems may develop.

During adulthood, the person may experience infertility, hypogonadism, and sparse pubic hair. The individual may develop diabetes. He or she is at risk for learning disabilities and attention deficit disorders. Some researchers have found children with PWS to have an unusual profile. They are strong in visual organization, including reading and vocabulary, but their spoken language is usually very poor. Auditory processing is poor, as are mathematics and writing skills.

HOW IS IT DIAGNOSED?

The genetics of PWS is very complicated and cannot be diagnosed with one simple test. Usually observation of some of the symptoms, such as poor muscle tone and sucking problems, is an initial clue. A specific test called DNA-based methylation can confirm the diagnosis in about 97 percent of cases. Because of the appearance of children, many cases are misdiagnosed as Down syndrome.

WHAT IS THE TREATMENT?

PWS has no cure, but there are several strategies to help manage the disorder. One of the first symptoms—that of difficulty sucking—can be treated with certain modification to nipples. When the lack of muscle tone is noted, hormone therapy may be given to increase tone, lean body mass, and movement.

When overeating begins between the ages of two to four, strict supervision is essential. Height and weight must be measured every six months. As the child gets older, the overweight and overeating are the biggest problems associated with this syndrome. Strategies may include locking cabinets and refrigerator. Gastric bypass and other surgical methods have not been successful with PWS.

Many other manifestations of the syndrome can be managed. For intellectual development, early intervention and behavioral therapy with strict guidelines can alleviate many of the problems related to this disorder. One persistent problem experienced by people with PWS is the high threshold to pain. They may experience intestinal, gall bladder, or appendicitis without being aware of it. Watching for symptoms is essential.

Other problems such as obstructive sleep apnea, curvature of the spine, eye problems, and sexual development issues may be helped by physician specialists.

For Further Information
Whittington, Joyce, and Tony Holland. *Prader-Willi Syndrome: Development and Manifestation*. New York: Cambridge University Press, 2011.

Progeria: Old at Eight

- Also known as Hutchinson-Gilford syndrome
- Rare; only 130 known cases worldwide since 1886
- Genetic disorder in which the child begins to age rapidly
- Average life expectancy is 13 years

Progeria, also called Hutchinson-Gilford syndrome, is a rare genetic disorder in which the child begins to age rapidly. The child develops many of the diseases and disorders connected with aging. Although the disorder is uncommon, the study of people with progeria has become important, in that it is leading to an understanding of the aging process. If we were listing the top 10 unusual diseases and disorders instead of 101, progeria would definitely be on that list.

WHAT IS PROGERIA?

Children with progeria appear normal at birth, but at some point within their first year, they begin to show signs that are not normal, and are associated with aging. Some of these signs include wrinkled and aging skin, loss of body fat and hair, and failure to thrive. The children look very similar despite different family characteristics and ethnic backgrounds. The disease is always fatal. The children die of heart attacks or strokes at about 13 years of age.

In 1886 Dr. Jonathan A. Hutchinson (1828–1913), a British physician, had a six-year-old boy brought into his office, who looked like a very old man. In a medical journal, he described how the boy not only looked old but that his organs were like that of a very old person. Several years later in 1897, Dr. Hastings Gilford (1861–1941), also a British physician, wrote about another boy with a similar condition and provided photographs of the progression of the boy's appearance over a number of years. The doctors used the term "progeria," a word that comes from two Greek roots: *pro,* meaning "before" and *geras,* meaning "old age." The word gerontology, which is the study of the aging process, comes from the same root word. Because of their interest and pioneer work in the disorder, the condition was named after the two: Hutchinson-Gilford Progeria Syndrome or HGPS.

Progeria is caused by a mutation in the *LMNA* or lamin A/C gene. The normal gene produces a protein that is responsible for the scaffold that holds the nucleus of the cell together. However, only one exchange in the amino acid bases that make up the structure can change the normal version of lamin A to an abnormal version. The mutation's replacing thymine for cytosine creates an abnormal protein called progerin, which in turn causes 50 amino acids at the telomere or end of the gene to drop off. The abnormal gene is then used in the cells to make the shape of the covering or envelope that covers the nucleus. Over time, this mutant process leads to an unstable nucleus, which in time produces the symptoms of progeria.

The gene responsible for progeria was isolated in April 2003, and reported in the journal *Nature*. It was found to be located on the long arm (q) of chromosome 1 at position 22. Although it can be inherited in a dominant pattern, most cases develop spontaneously, because the children die before they are old enough to pass the genes on to any offspring.

WHAT ARE THE SIGNS AND SYMPTOMS?

Although the child appears normal at birth, the developing symptoms follow a similar pattern.

- First, the physician may note a pattern of growth failure. The child does not gain weight.
- The skin begins to look very thin because of the loss of body fat; veins may show through the skin.
- The skin appears wrinkled and deposits of brown spots, the chemical lipofuscin, appear. The spots are prominent on hands and face of older adults.
- The face has a distinct look: eyes become prominent, nose appears like a beak at the tip, chin is small and protruding; ears tend to protrude. The children look very much like one another, though they are not related.
- Hair is lost, and the child becomes bald, a condition known as alopecia.
- Skeletal problems develop. The child may develop arthritis-like joints and osteoporosis.
- Diseases associated with aging develop. Arteriosclerosis or hardening of arteries to both the brain and heart appears.
- Other organs such as the kidneys, brain, adrenal glands, liver, and testes are affected.
- Death occurs as organs shut down.

However, some of the common conditions associated with aging are not present. The children do not develop cataracts, cancer, tumors, or senility. They still possess the ability to think, talk, learn, and communicate.

HOW IS IT DIAGNOSED?

Scientists supported by the Progeria Research Foundation have developed a diagnostic program that identifies the gene causing Progeria.

WHAT IS THE TREATMENT?

At this writing, a drug called farnesyltransferase inhibitor or FTI is in trials for potential treatment. However, until a cure is found, the children can be treated for the various symptoms that may extend their lives. Treating abnormal heart conditions with statins may extend their lives. Skeletal disorders may also be treated with drugs or physical therapy. When the insulating fat pads on the bottom of the feet become thin and cause pain, adding special soles to the shoes may alleviate the discomfort. Regular school is recommended, although certain physical accommodations may be needed.

CASE HISTORY: SAM'S STORY

Many children with the progeria disorder get little attention. They are born, live to their teen years, and die of heart disease at an average age of 13.

But Sam Bern's life was a different. He was born to two determined doctors, Leslie Gordon and Scott Berns, who encouraged Sam to tell his story through media and public speaking. When he was diagnosed in 1998 with this rare disease, his mother redirected her medical career and devoted all her time to working with Sam, and to developing the nonprofit Progeria Research Foundation. Sam's family has continued to lead the fight against progeria for more than 10 years, and was featured in an HBO documentary called *Life According to Sam*. In 2003, the Progeria Research Foundation supported efforts to find the gene that causes this disorder, which in turn has led to a drug that at this writing, is in trials.

Sam developed into an energetic boy, who in spite of the strikes against him, became a celebrity in his own right. He developed his interests in games like most boys, and was a good student at Foxborough Massachusetts High School. He was in the marching band, and played a snare drum especially designed for his 50-pound frame. He even attended his high school prom. But most of all he stayed positive, and kept his head up.

One of his favorite activities was going to the games of his favorite team—the New England Patriots. On Saturday night, January 11, 2014, the fans at Gillette Stadium in Boston planned to recognize Sam by making him an honorary captain. It was the playoff with the Indianapolis Colts. However, Sam died the night before the big game; he had succumbed to the aging syndrome after fighting it for 17 years. He had outlived the average of 13 years.

For Further Information

Okines, Hayley, and Kerry Okines. *Old Before My Time: Hayley Okines' Life with Progeria.* Columbia, MO: Accent Press, 2012.

Progeria Research Foundation: www.progeriaresearch.org

Prognathism: The Jaw That Brought Down a Dynasty

- A dominant inherited condition
- Appears as a thick lower lip, jutting jaw, and enlarged tongue
- Can cause problems with chewing, eating, and speaking
- Can be corrected today with dental and facial surgery

For four centuries, the Habsburg family ruled the thrones of Europe. It was a very powerful family, and although they had strong armies, they also had arranged marriages and intermarriages to keep the family secure politically. The intermarriage was their ultimate downfall. The condition that most typifies the family is called the Habsburg jaw. (See sidebar.) The jaw is an example of mandibular prognathism.

This disorder is well known in the history of genetics, but is still present today in some individuals.

WHAT IS PROGNATHISM?

Prognathism is one of the best-known examples of a facial genetic trait in humans. Normally, the lower jaw or jawbone or mandible is the moveable part of the mouth. The upper jaw or maxilla is created when two bones come together, securing the upper row of teeth. The protuberance at the back part of the mandible is called the condylar head. Where the two join together is the temporomandibular joint (TMJ), the hinge joint between the mandible and the temporal bone. When teeth fit together and function properly, it is called occlusion.

When the position of the maxilla and mandible do not come together or align, it is called malocclusion. In mandibular prognathism, the lower incisors and upper incisors overlap, the jaw protrudes, and the face is disfigured. The word prognathism comes from two Greek roots: *pro* meaning "forward," and *gnathos* meaning "jaw." The individual's top teeth and lower teeth do not align properly.

Mandibular prognathism is one of the types of prognathism and the most common. There are other types of prognathism that can be a symptom of other syndromes or conditions. For example, if the upper part of the jaw, the maxilla, the person may have maxillary prognathism. This condition may be commonly referred to as "buck-toothed" because the front teeth may protrude. Another condition, bimaxillary prognathism, may occur with both jaws stick out further than the face.

Several other genetic disorders may cause prognathism. These include acromegaly, a condition when the body produces too much growth hormone and the lower jaw sticks out as it becomes larger. Some rare genetic conditions, such as basal cell nevus syndrome, cause abnormal facial characteristics, including the jutting jaw.

WHAT ARE THE SIGNS AND SYMPTOMS?

The protrusion of the lower jaw is the obvious symptom. The lower jaw extends in front of the upper jaw, pushing it forward. The person can close the teeth and move the lower teeth to cover the upper front teeth. The lips and tongue may appear thick. The face may also appear long in some persons.

Although this condition is of major concern to humans, other animals also have the condition. Several of the great apes have prognathism. Also, certain breeds of dogs such as boxers and shih tzus are well known for their protruding jaws.

At birth, the extended jaw can be part of a normal face shape, but this shape may correct as the child gets older and teeth come in. In prognathism, the development of the mandible appears to be related to excessive growth of the condylar head (the protruding area at the back of the jaw bone) and the temporomandibular joint. A single dominant gene is thought to cause the disorder.

HOW IS IT DIAGNOSED?

The doctor may perform a physical examination and ask about family history of unusual jaw shapes, or difficulty in talking, biting, or chewing. The person will

---

HOW GENETICS CHANGED HISTORY

The House of Habsburg was one of the most powerful Royal Houses of Europe. They occupied the throne of the Holy Roman Empire from 1438 until 1740. Their relatives were everywhere. They produced emperors and kings who ruled Bohemia, England, France, Germany, Hungary, Russia, Croatia, the Second Mexican Empire, Ireland, Portugal, and Spain, as well as rulers of Dutch and Italian principalities.

Their strong belief was that the best spouse for a Habsburg was another Habsburg. Thus, marriages were arranged between first cousins, or between uncle and niece. A study of 3,000 members of the family over 16 generations suggests that inbreeding directly led to their extinction.

Follow a group of portraits or statues of the Habsburgs, and it is easily traceable through the family. In the 15th century, a female from a Polish family from Masovia married Duke Ernest of Inner Austria, a member of the Habsburg family. The defect is seen on sculptures of tombs of the ruling family of the ancestors of this woman at St. John's Cathedral in Warsaw. Maximilian I in 1519 sent the gene to both Spanish and Austrian lines for two centuries, by marrying his son Philip II (the Handsome) to the Spanish queen Joanna of Castile, and set it up for his grandson Charles (Carlos) to be ruler of Spain and to succeed him as Holy Roman Emperor.

A famous painting of Maximilian by Albrecht Durer shows the prominence of the jaw. Leopold I (1658-1705) of Austria had a coin issued with his picture, which the people referred to as Leopold the Hog Mouth. He had the prominent jaw and large lips.

Victor McKusick (1921–2008), a well-known medical geneticist, traced 13 families with Habsburg marriages with 409 members and 23 generations. Over time, it showed how royal inbreeding passed on the trait, which became exaggerated over time. Charles II (Carlos) of Spain was the result of multiple marriages of cousins. He was physical and intellectually disabled and disfigured. He had a large tongue, which made it difficult to understand his speech. He had two wives but was impotent, and left no heirs. The 16 generations of inbreeding left Charles II with a genome similar to that of the offspring of a brother and sister.

then be referred to a dental specialist who will take skull x-rays, dental x-rays, and imprints of the bite using a plaster mold of the teeth.

WHAT IS THE TREATMENT?

Surgery is probably essential for treatment of the malocclusion of the teeth and bones. If the teeth are overcrowded, extraction and braces may begin the year-long process. Then dental specialists will perform a process called orthognathic surgery that will modify the jaw and remove part of the mandible. This procedure allows the jawbone to be aligned using screws and plates. Another year of orthodontic treatment follows.

For Further Information

Chudley, Albert E. "Genetic Landmarks through Philately: The Habsburg Jaw." *Clinical Genetics* 54 (4): 283–4, 1998.

Uncombable Hair Syndrome: Hair Like Spun Glass

- Rare; less than 100 cases reported in medical journals since 1973
- Autosomal dominant condition
- Hair is unruly and cannot be controlled by combing and brushing
- Treatment in children not usually successful; person may outgrow some of the difficulties

If you have ever tried to put angel hair on a holiday tree, you can picture this syndrome. Angel hair is made from very thin spun glass, and is completely uncontrollable. This is what uncombable hair syndrome resembles. The hair sticks straight out from the scalp and cannot be combed flat. No amount of brushing or combing controls it.

WHAT IS UNCOMBABLE HAIR SYNDROME?

Uncombable hair syndrome is a condition in which the hair stands straight up from the scalp in an unruly pattern and cannot be managed by combing or brushing.

Although uncombable hair syndrome was only recognized in the 20th century, German folk tales talked about children with unruly hair for over 150 years. In 1845 a German doctor wrote a morality tale called *Der Struwwelpeter* (slovenly or shaggy Peter) about a naughty boy with unruly blonde hair and long nails. The boy with unruly hair refused to groom himself. The story was based on old folk tales about children with wild hair who were thought to have wild behavior. Two French doctors described a possible case of uncombable hair in 1912 in their book *Les Velus*, which included a syndrome they called "chevelure en vadrouille" or mop hair. The hair reminded them of the mop that sailors used to scrub the decks of a ship. Later in 1972, three French doctors named it *cheveux incoiffables* meaning "uncontrollable hair." Later that same year independent American researchers J. D. Stroud and A. H. Mehregan, gave it the picturesque name, the "spun-glass hair syndrome."

With normal hair structure, each hair grows out of its single live sac called a follicle, which is located in the subcutaneous tissue of the scalp. There, the hair root gets nourishment from tiny capillaries that surround it. From that root a shaft extends to the surface. The hair itself is made of the dead protein keratin, the same protein as the outer layer of the skin. The shape of the shaft determines the nature of the hair. If the shaft is round, the hair is straight; if the shaft is flat, the hair is curly. Those with wavy hair have an oval shaft. A cross-section of the hair shaft of a person with uncombable hair syndrome under the electron microscope reveals that the shaft is kidney-shaped, or like a triangle. Another theory of the cause is that the hair may form prematurely in the shaft. To be noticeable, over 50 percent of the hairs must be affected by the abnormal structure of the hair shaft.

Uncombable hair syndrome is considered to be an autosomal dominant condition, in which one parent has the gene or condition. Garty et al. in a 1982 *Archives of Disease in Childhood* article, reported a case of a little boy whose hair could not be combed. The boy's father had similar hair, but the father's hair had become normal at about the age of five. The boy's grandfather and great-grandfather were said to have had the same hair in infancy. In addition, 12 boys and 15 girls related to the family had the same unruly hair. Most cases improved with the onset of puberty.

WHAT ARE THE SIGNS AND SYMPTOMS

The hair on the head stands straight up and cannot be managed with brushing or combing, which may lead to tangles or mats. The condition appears to be noticeable between three months to 12 years of age. The hair is not unusually thick or thin and is normal in quantity. However, the color may different from other members of the family in that it is usually silver, blonde, or straw colored. Eyebrows and eyelashes are normal.

HOW IS IT DIAGNOSED?

Usually just a look at the hair can determine the syndrome. Examination of cross sections of the scalp embedded in paraffin can determine the triangular or kidney-shaped cross section.

WHAT IS THE TREATMENT?

Treatment in children is not usually successful. Researchers have tried some different things with limited success. Some cases of uncombable hair can be treated with biotin, also known as vitamin H. Use of shampoo with zinc pyrithione and conditioners may help moisturize the hair and give an element of control. Lubricating hair products that have other moisturizers may also help revive some of the tangling and wild tendencies. There is usually hope for improvement as the child ages. One study points out that it may be abnormal in infancy and early childhood, but will improve with the years.

For Further Information

Hicks, J., D. W. Metry, J. Barrish, and M. Levy. "Uncombable Hair (Cheveux Incoiffables, Pili Trianguli et Canaliculi) Syndrome: Brief Review and Role of Scanning Electron Microscopy in Diagnosis." *Ultrastruct Pathol* 25 (2): 99–103, 2001.

PART II

UNUSUAL MENTAL HEALTH DISORDERS

WHAT YOU SHOULD KNOW ABOUT MENTAL HEALTH DISORDERS

Some of these disorders you may know or have heard of, such as kleptomania, but you probably know little other than the name, and that these people steal not for any gain, but from an innate urge; the items taken have little or no value.

You also may not know many of the disorders by their official name. Such disorders as hybristophilia, women who fall in love with serial killers, or erotomania, people who fall in love with some celebrity and do things to pursue them, are two commonly known conditions that people have heard of, while unaware of their official names. An example of a person with erotomania is John Hinckley, who shot President Reagan to impress actor Jodie Foster.

Others were chosen because of their usual manifestations, such as alien hand syndrome. Or Capgras delusion, demonstrated by people who think their loved ones have been replaced by imposters. Munchausen syndrome is a condition in which people fake illness to get attention, and may actually hurt or mutilate themselves to get admitted to a health care facility.

The guidelines for most mental health disorders are found in *The Diagnostic and Statistical Manual of Mental Disorders* (*DSM*), published by the American Psychiatric Association. This manual seeks to standardize the criteria and language for clinicians, researchers, and others. *DSM* is now in its fifth edition, which was published in May 2013. The World Health Organization also lists disorders in the International Statistical Classification of Diseases and Related Health Problems, 10th revision (ICD-10).

Many interesting conditions could have been chosen, but these 19 were considered examples of different kinds of illnesses. Most of the causes and treatments for these disorders are controversial; therefore, the treatment section for these disorders is generally shorter than the symptoms section.

For Further Information

American Psychiatric Association. *Diagnostic and Statistical Manual of Mental Disorders*, 5th ed. American Psychiatric Association, 2013.

National Institute of Mental Health: http://www.nimh.nih.gov.

Noll, Richard. *Bizarre Diseases of the Mind*. New York: Berkley, 1990.

Sacks, Oliver. *Hallucinations*. London: Pan MacMillan UK, 2012.

Alien Hand Syndrome: When the Right Hand Does Not Know What the Left Is Doing

- Also known as Dr. Strangelove Syndrome, capricious hand, anarchic hand
- Person has feeling in his or her hand, but is unable to control the movements
- The hand appears to have a mind of its own
- May be related to damage of the corpus callosum

In the movie *Dr. Strangelove*, the title character in the movie has a strange affliction. Strangelove is a former Nazi. In the movie he struggles to keep his right arm from giving the Nazi salute. The hand has a mind of its own and has to be restrained. The movie, which was a comedy spoof on the cold war, featured Peter Sellers, who plays this character and two other roles. Many people watching Strangelove's ordeal with his hand thought it was extremely funny and never suspected that he was portraying someone with a rare, neurological problem—alien hand syndrome. At first glance, alien hand syndrome sounds impossible, but although it is rare, it is a real syndrome with physical and mental ramifications.

The cause of the syndrome is not exactly known, and may depend on the circumstances. If the corpus callosum (the area connecting the two hemispheres) is damaged, the person's nondominant hand may counteract the movement of the dominant hand. For example, one hand pushes a chair forward while the other one pulls it back. This counteractive movement is one of the most common. Some physicians have reported an instance in which a person will button a shirt with one hand, and the other one will immediately unbutton. One man tore pieces of his clothes or other objects with his alien hand and was completely unaware of these movements; the other hand struggled to keep the hand from ripping the clothes.

Several areas of the brain may be affected. Damage to the frontal lobe can trigger reaching, grasping, or movements in the opposite hand. For example, one person with the damage to the frontal lobe might grasp something but not release it. The voluntary hand may have to peel the fingers off to let go of the object. If the back of the brain is damaged, the person may lift the hand in the air and the other will withdraw it. A mirror reaction may occur if the person voluntarily moves the hand away from the body, the alien hand will move away from the body in the opposite direction.

WHAT IS ALIEN HAND SYNDROME?

In alien hand syndrome, the person's hand moves involuntarily and acts independently of the other hand. Sometimes the hand moves in contrast with the intent of the other hand. The symptoms are brought about through some injury or secondary insult to the brain. Causes include stroke, trauma, tumor, surgery, or some type of degenerative brain condition, such as Alzheimer's or Creutzfeldt-Jakob disease.

In order to understand alien hand syndrome, one must first understand the anatomy of the brain. The brain weighs about two pounds and is made of two hemispheres. It might be likened to the appearance of a whole shelled walnut; you can see two halves called the right and left hemispheres. The two sides are joined by a tough network band of nerves called the corpus callosum. The front part of both hemispheres is called the frontal lobe; the areas at the top are the parietal lobes and those at the back are the occipital region. Injury to these distinct parts can cause the various symptoms of alien hand syndrome.

In 1908, Kurt Goldstein (1878–1965), a German psychiatrist, first encountered a woman who had suffered a stroke that had paralyzed the left side of the body. She was right-handed and felt that her left arm belonged to another person, because it performed things she did not want it to. Goldstein was the first to observe alien hand, and several other disconnection syndromes associated with brain anatomy. In 1972, Norman Geschwind (1926–1984), who was also known for his exploration of behavioral neurology based on analysis of lesions in the brain, later defined the disorder.

WHAT ARE THE SIGNS AND SYMPTOMS?

A person with this syndrome feels normal sensations but in his mind believes that the hand behaves differently from the behavior that the person wants. Depending upon the nature of the injury and the part of the brain affected, the movements may be random or purposeful, and can affect the dominant or nondominant hand. There are several subtypes of symptoms.

HOW IS IT DIAGNOSED?

The person who is experiencing the alien hand can tell his or her physician about it, and the physician can possibly observe the alien hand in action. Studying which area of the brain is damaged can be done with a technique called functional magnetic resonance imaging (fMRI). The brain scan can be done while the person is sitting. If the hand moves, brain activity in several areas can be observed.

WHAT IS THE TREATMENT?

There is no cure. There are some types of restraints that may be put on the alien hand. One strategy might be to give that hand something to do or to hold, such as a cane. Another strategy might be to muff the hand with a soft hand glove or mitt. Theoretically, this would impede the involuntary movements of the hand.

For Further Information
Bellows, Alan. *Alien Hand Syndrome*. New York: Workman Publishing, 2009.

Androphobia: Fear of Men

- A rare disorder in which the person has an inordinate fear of men
- Symptoms resemble other panic disorders
- May be caused by early childhood trauma
- Not to be confused with misandry, hatred of men

To most, this disorder may appear exceedingly strange and bizarre. But it is a real phobia that a few women have, and can be devastating. Although some of the causes may lie in childhood, many factors play into the disorder. It should not be confused with the term "misandry," in which the person has a real dislike and even hatred of men, but does not show the psychological symptoms of androphobia.

Androphobia is one of many phobias that are listed in *The Diagnostic and Statistical Manual of Mental Disorders 5,* but is considered one of the rarest.

WHAT IS ANDROPHOBIA?

Androphobia comes from two Greek words *andras* meaning "man," and *phobos* meaning "fear." It is an intense and irrational fear of men. The person cannot explain the fear, but it leads him or her to avoid men whenever possible. The work life and personal life of the person is affected to a great extent. The person may have a normal life and make friends with girls and women, but will avoid men in all situations.

Finding the cause and diagnosing the condition is a challenge. The person may not admit that he or she has a problem, and try to hide it by only dealing with females. The causes may vary. Most psychiatrists think that there was some traumatic event or abuse that happened in the life of the person, or that he or she might have witnessed some terrible incident that involved men. However, some psychologists also believe that body chemistry and genetics play a part in developing the phobia.

WHAT ARE THE SIGNS AND SYMPTOMS?

The person with androphobia will have symptoms of a panic attack when he or she is around men. She may become dizzy, breathless, nauseous, and sweaty. The heart may begin to beat rapidly and his mouth will become dry. In the presence of men, he or she is unable to articulate words or sentences.

HOW IS IT DIAGNOSED?

This rare condition may be difficult to diagnose because those affected will make friends with many people, and live a somewhat normal life. The person may go for help because he or she feels sweaty or numb when around men. However, many people with the symptoms keep quiet out of embarrassment.

WHAT IS THE TREATMENT?

Scientists are trying to understand the nature of the large number of phobias, to help find causes and therapies. However, as with most treatments of phobias, it is not just trial and error. It is essential that the person be under the care of a qualified health care professional. The doctors will use several methods which include exposure therapy, meaning having the person face the fear, talk therapy, and relaxation therapy. The health care professionals also recommend that the person find a support group, which meets as a group regularly, or on line. The group therapy may help the person face the disorder. The last treatment is anti-anxiety medication, which is seldom used because of side effects.

For Further Information

Milosevic, Irena, and Randi McCabe. *Phobias: The Psychology of Irrational Fear*. Santa Barbara, CA: ABC-CLIO, 2015.

Bigorexia: When Muscles Are All That Matter

- Also known as muscle dysmorphia, megarexia, reverse anorexia nervosa, or Adonis complex
- A specific type of compulsion to build muscles according to a perceived image of the perfect male body
- Exact number of individuals affected is not known but some estimate that it is in the thousands
- Onset starts in late teens

In Greek mythology, Adonis is the half-man, half-god, who is the epitome of masculine beauty. He is so handsome that he wins the love of Aphrodite, the beauty queen of the gods. His masculinity was annually renewed, and he was ever youthful, strong, and appealing. The term "Adonis" is sometimes applied to handsome young men.

In her article "Adonis Complex: A Body Image Problem Facing Men and Boys," Natasha Tracy describes how the term "Adonis Complex" has been coined to describe a variety of body image concerns that have plagued boys and men, especially since the early 2000s. According to the author, these men are so preoccupied with body building that they jeopardize careers and relationships. The term "bigorexia" is used as a way of equating this obsession with the eating disorder anorexia nervosa. Bigorexia is to "huge" what anorexia is to "thin." In fact, it combines the word "big" with the Greek word *orexia,* meaning "appetite" in the sense of wanting something.

This serious mental disorder has developed in the last couple of decades and may still be unknown to most people. Attention has been paid to female eating disorders such as anorexia, but bigorexia is still largely unknown.

WHAT IS BIGOREXIA?

Bigorexia is the obsession with muscle development that is similar to anorexia. In this mental disorder, the man perceives himself to have inadequate muscles. Also called muscular dysmorphia, sociologist Anthony Cortese calls it an obsessive compulsive disorder that focuses on building muscles and attaining an unrealistic, idealized picture of the male body.

Muscular dysmorphia was coined in 1997 to describe the disorder; commonly, it is called bigorexia. The individuals are so obsessed that they may exercise through pain and broken bones, and lose their jobs rather than miss their training sessions. However, these men, who actually have a great physique, may really hate their bodies and think that they are not measuring up to what they should be.

The standards for male beauty are always changing. Mass culture bombards males with pictures of an idealized body. Movies and ads present idealized and unrealistic people, whom males then emulate and idolize.

WHAT ARE THE SIGNS AND SYMPTOMS?

People with bigorexia or muscle dysmorphia have a perception problem. They see themselves through a distorted lens of physical inadequacies. Their muscles may be bulging and sculpted, but no amount of persuasion can convince them that they are good enough. They then begin to hate their bodies and will not display them as a body builder might, but will wear baggy clothing to conceal their bodies. The discouragement may also lead to depression.

The symptoms are outlined in the *Diagnostic and Statistical Manual of Mental Disorders 5.* The person may be so obsessed that he looks at his body in the mirror, sometimes as many as 50 times a day. He may think about his body often and consider that he must be leaner and more muscular. The person may eat special high protein, low fat diets that promise to help him gain muscle; he may refuse to eat out because he has no control over the exact amount of food. The person may train when injured because he cannot afford to lose muscle. He may also turn down social events, skip family gatherings, or neglect job responsibilities.

Some of the individuals take anabolic steroids. Although they may know that long-term use may damage liver, heart, muscles, and cause acne, they still persist. Steroid use can raise cholesterol and develop breasts. The most egregious side effect of steroids is mood swings, anger, and rage. The common misperception is that when they are prescribed by a doctor, they are safe.

Men with bigorexia may have low self-esteem. Some report having been teased about their physique in school, and determining to do something about it when they got older. However, they never seem to attain that picture of the ideal body that is in their minds. One study in 2000 found that over 29 percent of these men had a history of anxiety disorder, and 50 percent had some type of mood disorder. Bigorexia can be found in women, but generally this is rare.

HOW IS IT DIAGNOSED?

Several theories try to explain. One called cognitive theory searches for causes of the negative appraisal and dysfunctional thoughts about the body image. The psychodynamic theory seeks to find troubling thoughts from childhood that lead to emotional conflict. The cognitive-behavioral theory combines culture with psychological problems, such as low self-esteem due to childhood experiences such as bullying or teasing. A biological theory traces the idea to chemical imbalances, such as serotonin irregularity.

WHAT IS THE TREATMENT?

Most men with the disorder will not admit there is a problem, and therefore make treatment quite difficult. There really have been no effective studies of those who have come forward and been diagnosed with the problem. If the person does realize there is a problem, there are a number of options: cognitive-behavioral therapy that helps identify problems and changing patterns of thinking to be more realistic, psychodynamic therapy, or drugs used for other similar disorders.

For Further Information

Reel, Justine J. *Eating Disorders: An Encyclopedia of Causes, Treatment, and Prevention.* Santa Barbara, CA: ABC-CLIO, 2013.

Capgras Delusion: A Body Snatcher Is in My House

- Very rare; more women than men appear to have the condition
- Person believes an imposter has taken over the body of another
- The "imposter" is a key person in that individual's life
- Some researchers believe there is an organic cause

In 1956 a film called *Invasion of the Body Snatchers* was popular with moviegoers. The story told of a California town in which members of the community were convinced impostors had invaded the bodies of their friends and relatives. Of course, in the movie, aliens were attacking the community by taking over real bodies. This theme of the invading aliens is popular in science fiction movies. But with Capgras delusion, it is quite real to the person experiencing it.

Capgras delusion is a condition in which the person thinks an impostor has taken over the body of someone he or she knows. The delusion, which is unusual, was at first thought a psychosis; however, some new evidence, of a neurological basis that occurred as some type of brain injury, does exist.

WHAT IS CAPGRAS DELUSION?

Capgras delusion (pronounced *kapp*-grah) is a rare disorder in which a person is convinced that someone has been replaced by another individual or being. The replaced person may be a spouse, parent, family member, or friend. The impostor looks exactly like the person, but in the mind of the perceiver is not that person. The syndrome is known as a delusional misidentification.

Jean Marie Joseph Capgras (1873–1950), a French psychiatrist, first described this disorder in 1923. Along with Jean Reboul-Lachaux, he told of a patient, Madame M., who told him that impostors had taken over the bodies of her friends and family. According to Madame M., 80 different impostors had taken over her husband's body, one at a time. In a paper published in a French medical journal, Capgras and Reboul-Lachaux called the condition *l'illusion des sosies*, which means "the illusion of look-alikes." Over the years, the illusion began to bear Capgras's name.

Since the 1980s, most researchers believe that there is an organic cause, which is caused by chemical or physical changes to the brain. The causes could be from a stroke, drug overdose, accidents that damaged the right side of the brain, or other diseases.

WHAT ARE THE SIGNS AND SYMPTOMS?

The delusion that the person is experiencing is not a hallucination, which is something that one's senses feel, that is not actually real. Delusions are related to a person's thoughts. The person actually believes something exists that is not true. Following are the characteristics of the delusion:

- The individual is truly convinced that one or several persons have been replaced by an impostor.
- The person sees others as real but perceives them as doubles.
- The delusion may also extend to animals or inanimate objects.
- The person is aware that these perceptions are abnormal; they are not hallucinating.
- The supposed impostor is usually a key figure in the life of a person, usually a spouse.

Carol Berman, a psychiatrist at New York University Medical Center, recalls a 37-year-old woman who came into her office complaining that she returned to her house to find a strange man sitting on her couch. He was wearing her husband's clothes, but he did not look right. She was convinced the man was an imposter.

V. S. Ramachandran, a neuroscientist at the University of California, San Diego, told of a student who was severely injured in a car accident. He was in a coma for several weeks, then appeared to be doing fine. However, when his mother came in to see him, he said that this woman looked like his mother, but was not. She was an imposter.

HOW IS IT DIAGNOSED?

At one time, the delusion was diagnosed with a Freudian psychoanalytic approach. The person had some sexual desire or repressed feelings and was resolving guilt in this manner. It was especially diagnosed in middle-aged women who were thought to have hysteria. This psychodynamic theory has generally been discredited and replaced by thinking that something is actually physically wrong in the brain. J. R. Benson, in a 1983 issue of *American Journal of Psychiatry*, presented a review of 133 cases of Capgras delusion, and suggested that the causes were physical.

The person may be diagnosed to have other disorders that also affect the brain, such as schizophrenia, Huntington disease, multiple sclerosis, and dementia. Persons with Alzheimer's disease, a disorder in which plaque deposits affect the neurotransmitters in the brain, appear to have these delusions often. Drug use may lead to the disorder. The person may be taking drugs, and experiencing substance-induced delusional disorders. Mood disorders with delusions such as manic or depressive types may also be related. In fact, today Capgras syndrome is basically understood as a neurological disorder with some type of brain injury or degeneration.

WHAT IS THE TREATMENT?

Because the delusions are so individual, the treatment likewise must be individual. Some people, who have no other problems, may recover on their own. The San Diego male student described by Ramachandran eventually recovered. Patients with other mental disorder may be helped with medication. Antipsychotic drugs, such as pimozide, risperdone, or clopazine, have been used with some success. Counseling, using reality testing and reframing, must be used with care, because the person is really convinced the impostor is real.

For Further Information
Vaknin, Sam. *The Capgras Shift.* Rhinebeck, NY: Narcissus Publications, 2011.

Cotard Syndrome: The Walking Dead

- A neurological and/or psychiatric condition in which the person thinks he or she is dead or that a body part is dead or missing
- People with the syndrome often withdraw from the world
- Not classified in any edition of the *Diagnostic and Statistical Manual of Mental Disorders*, but may be associated with some psychiatric conditions
- As of 2013, there have been over 1,000 documented cases in the literature

In 2005, a 32-year-old Iranian man arrived at a hospital claiming that he was dead and had been turned into a dog. He believed that his relatives had tried to poison him, but that God had protected him. He was diagnosed with Cotard syndrome and treated with electro-convulsive therapy, which relieved his major symptoms. Because of its unusual manifestations, Cotard syndrome excites imagination and interest. The TV show *Scrubs* had an episode in which a male patient believes that he is dead.

WHAT IS COTARD SYNDROME?

Cotard syndrome or delusion is a rare condition in which people think they are dead, and are walking corpses. Some believe that they already have died, or that their blood, organs, or limbs are dead and decaying. Although it is more common in middle-aged or older females, people of either sex and at any age may have this neuropsychiatric syndrome. In a few documented cases, a younger person has been diagnosed. One of the youngest patients was a 14-year-old boy with epilepsy who was convinced that he and everyone else was dead, including all the trees.

In 1788 Charles Bonnet (1720–1793), a philosopher and doctor who resided in Switzerland, encountered an older woman who thought she was dead, and who demanded that her family put her in a shroud and place her in a coffin. During her "wake" she complained that the shroud was not the right color and that it was not fixed properly. She was treated with a "powder of precious stones and opium," which relieved her symptoms for a short period of time.

About 100 years later, Jules Cotard (1840–1889), a French neurologist, saw Mademoiselle X, who claimed to have no brain, no stomach, and no intestines. Because she had no vital organs, she believed that she was immortal and refused to eat. In 1880, Cotard gave a lecture in Paris about the symptoms of the syndrome, which ranged from mild to severe. Interest in the case spread widely, and the disorder was given his name.

Several explanations exist for Cotard syndrome. Many of the cases are associated with other psychiatric disorders, such as bipolar depression or schizophrenia. A second explanation is that neurological problems caused by trauma or other conditions causes the brain to atrophy, and results in the delusion. A 1986 article in the *Journal of Clinical Psychiatry* describes lesions in the parietal lobe of the brain, and atrophy in the frontal lobe of patients. One study using PET scans showed low metabolism activity in the brain. Researchers found that large areas of the frontal and parietal brain had almost no activity, and compared it to that of people in a vegetative state.

WHAT ARE THE SIGNS AND SYMPTOMS?

The term "negation," meaning that the person has ceased to exist, describes the core symptom of Cotard. The person believes that he or she does not exist as a human being, and is therefore a walking corpse. In 2007, Yarnada, et al. in a Scandinavian psychiatric journal described three distinct stages of the syndrome:

- **Germination.** The person exhibits some signs of depression and belief that he or she is ill (hypochondria).
- **Blooming.** The person begins to think that he does not exist and eventually develops the full-blown attributes of the syndrome.
- **Chronic.** Now the delusions are severe, and depression is overwhelming.

The most obvious symptom is the distortion of reality. For example, in 1996, a young man in Edinburgh had a brain injury as a result of a motorcycle accident.

Although he recovered from the accident, he believed that he had died of complications from it. He and his mother soon moved to South Africa. Because of the heat, he was convinced that he had been taken to hell and that he really was dead.

Because they believe they are already dead, persons with Cotard may do things that would cause serious bodily injury. They may kill themselves by doing daring feats s such as flying like a bird. Because they believe they are dead, they may refuse to eat or drink, and may starve themselves to death.

HOW IS IT DIAGNOSED?

This disorder is not listed as a separate syndrome in any edition of the *Diagnostic and Statistical Manual of Mental Disorders,* the guiding text for diagnosing mental diseases in the United States. However, it does have an International Classification of Diseases (ICD) code for listing in Europe.

WHAT IS THE TREATMENT?

Some pharmacological intervention may be used. Several types of antidepressants, antipsychotics, and mood stabilizers may be used. Others have been treated with electroshock therapy.

For Further Information

Berrios, G. E. and R. Luque. "Cotard Syndrome: Clinical Analysis of 100 Cases." *Acta Psychiatrica Scandinavica* 91 (March 1995):185–188.

Diogenes Syndrome: A Messy House Can Be Life-Threatening

- Behavioral disorder exhibited by people who prefer to live in squalor
- May be related to other mental disorders
- May be the result of injury to the frontal lobe of the brain
- People with the syndrome refuse help

Diogenes was a Greek philosopher who lived in the fourth century BCE, and believed in complete self-sufficiency. He was a true cynic regarding society and its accumulation of material things. He rejected these ideas, and lived in a large clay jar in Athens. He did go into the Agora (the public marketplace) to debate people and present his theories of living. A. N. G. Clarke et al. in the mid-1970s, named the syndrome "Diogenes" after the lifestyle exhibited by the philosopher. However, the application of Diogenes's name is used more in the popular media and articles; geriatricians and psychiatrists use the name sparingly, preferring to use one of the other names. A typical case history is presented and paraphrased from the journal *Clinical Geriatrics*.

The person who displays Diogenes syndrome lives in an unusual environment but does not have a mental disorder.

WHAT IS DIOGENES SYNDROME?

Diogenes syndrome is a behavioral disorder exhibited by some older adults who neglect their surroundings, their hygiene, and personal health. The person may also exhibit compulsive hoarding and social withdrawal, but with no shame about it. The term is used more in popular media and briefly mentioned by those who work in gerontology or psychiatry.

The disorder may be divided into two types:

1. Primary—The person is highly intelligent but aggressive, stubborn, suspicious, emotionally unstable, and has an unreal perception of life.
2. Secondary—The condition is related to mental disorders.

Several theories of the cause are presented. However, none of the theories appear to relate to poverty in early life or to traumatic childhood experiences. Following are some of the suggested causes:

- Researchers D. Macmillan and P. Shaw (1966) in an article in the *British Medical Journal* suggested that senile breakdown in the standards of personal and environmental cleanliness is a syndrome.
- A. N. Clarke (1975) in the medical journal *The Lancet* suggested that the person seeks self-sufficiency and freedom from social constraint and material values, and named these attributes after Diogenes. He related these behaviors to stress-related defense mechanisms of the elderly, and possibly to the natural aging process.
- Post (1982) applied the term "senile recluse" and proposed that this was the end stage of a personality disorder of people who are aloof, domineering, suspicious, aggressive, and obstinate.
- Some psychologists explain this as obsessive-compulsive disorder or obsessive-compulsive personality; however, Diogenes syndrome is not listed in any of the DSM manuals.
- Many of those affected were raised during the depression when their families had very little. This action may explain the hoarding tendency. Some features of

the disorder also correspond with a diagnosis of dementia, cognitive disability, schizophrenia, delusional disorder, and personality disorders, but these generally are not thought to be Diogenes syndrome.

- A more current idea suggests that these people have suffered an injury to the frontal lobe of the brain. The frontal lobes are the areas involved in the higher order thinking processes, including reasoning and decision making.

WHAT ARE THE SIGNS AND SYMPTOMS?

People with the syndrome experience social isolation. The person, who is usually above normal intelligence, begins to ignore his surroundings, allowing trash and other things that they are hoarding to accumulate. They ignore their personal hygiene and may refuse help. Following are the attributes of those with Diogenes syndrome:

- They choose to live in unsanitary conditions and are comfortable in those situations.
- They have a distorted sense of reality and have no shame about their living conditions.
- They may suffer from unpredictable mood swings and are aggressive, stubborn, and suspicious of others.
- They suffer from nutritional deficiencies and other health-related problems.

Nearly all of those designated with this syndrome have above-average intelligence and have had stable and successful careers.

HOW IS IT DIAGNOSED?

Diagnosis of this condition is very difficult, because the person may refuse to accept any kind of help even when ordered by the courts. When treated in an institutional setting, the person may return to the old ways when going back to the home.

WHAT IS THE TREATMENT?

Management of people with Diogenes syndrome is very difficult. The main objectives of the health care professional is to help the individual improve the patent's lifestyle and well-being, so they must decide whether they can force this on the person. The personality of skepticism and cynicism makes them suspicious of any outside help. Some have found success in getting them to adult day care facilities. Other methods include services to the patient's home such as the delivery of food.

CASE HISTORY: MS. G.

From the outside of the apartment of Ms. G, a 72-year-old single white female, there was a terrible stench that took over the entire apartment complex. Neighbors contacted the local mental health services, who found carpets soaked with urine and moldy feces, five-feet high piles of garbage, and no furniture or refrigerator. The only evidence of food was piles of cracker wrappers.

Ms. G's physical appearance was in the same state of neglect. She had layers of dirty clothes stained with urine, and very dirty skin. She refused to communicate with the services and resisted any professional help. She was then put involuntarily into a geriatric psychiatric unit. She had several physical problems, but no sign of dementia, and her memory and cognitive functions were intact. She had no history of psychiatric illness. She did have a history of having no significant relationships with her relatives and no friends; that fact did not bother her.

She told the health professionals that she had a BS in sociology and worked as an employment counselor; however, she refused to give contact numbers and the facts could not be verified.

Ms. G. displayed all the typical characteristic of Diogenes syndrome. She strongly opposed her hospitalizations and declined all services. She was discharged from the hospital. They drew up a compliance plan, but she refused any follow-up care, and had no further contact with the hospital.

They may be committed to an institution for help but still refuse to accept any outside assistance. This is because they have no shame about their condition and do not think they are doing anything wrong. Results from hospitalization tend to be poor. Many die in the hospital.

For Further Information

Radebaugh, T. S., F. J. Hooper, and E. M. Gruenberg. "The Social Breakdown Syndrome in the Elderly Population Living in the Community: The Helping Study." *British Journal of Psychiatry* 151 (3): 341–6, 1987.

Dissociative Identity Disorder (DID): Multiple Personalities, One Body

- The term "multiple personalities" is no longer medically acceptable
- Prevalence: less than 1 percent of the general population
- Individual exhibits two or more distinct personalities, which "take over" the body at different times

- One of the most controversial psychiatric disorders, with no clear consensus on diagnosis or treatment

The idea that one individual can have two or even more distinct personalities is fascinating. Books about people who have one or more alters (alternate personalities) have piqued the interest of the public since they were first exposed to psychological ideas. In 1886, Scottish novelist Robert Louis Stevenson (1850–1894) wrote *The Strange Case of Dr. Jekyll and Mr. Hyde.* Dr. Jekyll was a well-respected physician and his alter personality was Mr. Hyde, a brutal killer. In 1957, the bestselling book *The Three Faces of Eve,* the story of Chris Costner Sizemore, excited the public about multiple personalities; in the years following the book and film, several cases of dissociative identity disorder (DID) were diagnosed. The most controversial book, *Sybil,* was published in 1974. The story of Shirley Ardell Mason helped popularize the diagnosis, but also introduced controversy regarding treatment.

Multiple personality disorders, now called dissociative identity disorders, are still controversial.

WHAT IS DISSOCIATIVE IDENTITY DISORDER?

Dissociative identity disorder is a condition in which one escapes reality in ways that are involuntary and that detach the person from what is happening in the world around them. At least two or more distinct personalities control the behavior or the individual.

At one time or another, most of us have daydreams or have escaped reality or boredom through imagination. Most people have also been lost in the moment when concentrating on a project. But that is part of one personality. Those with DID actually dissociate themselves and do not connect the memory, thoughts, feelings, or experiences of their different personalities. Each personality has its own separate identity, and the two or more are not connected, though they reside in the same body.

Some people may ask if DID is real. It is amazing that many personalities could develop in one person. Diagnosing it is challenging even for highly trained experts, and the condition itself remains controversial among those who have studied the disorder.

Ancient people were interested in behavior and believed that it was controlled by the humors and specific alignment of the stars. Greek physicians developed a system of medicine that posited four distinct bodily fluids determined the mental and physical health of a person. This system was help for centuries in medical thought. Paracelsus (1493–1541), the Swiss physician, brought a new approach of observation and experience to medicine; he described possibly the first case of DID in 1646. In the 18th century, Franz Mesmer (1734–1815) and others were pioneers of hypnosis; they were enchanted with the thought that during hypnosis two minds could exist. In the 19th century, the number of reported cases increased to about 100; during the latter part of that century, the idea that traumatic emotional experiences causes multiple personalities emerged.

Between 1880 and 1920, the whole idea of multiple personalities became a hot topic. Jean-Martin Charcot (1825–1893), known as the father of neurology and mentor of Sigmund Freud (1856–1939), identified Clara Norton Fowler as one of the first cases of DID to be scientifically studied. However, some of Charcot's work with hysteria was later discredited and exposed as fraudulent, causing disinterest in the pursuit of the diagnosis of multiple personalities. In the early years of the 20th century, interest continued to wane, when Eugen Bleuler (1857–1939) introduced the idea of schizophrenia, which then became the mental disease that drew a lot of attention.

In 1985, the third edition of *Diagnostic and Statistical Manual of Mental Disorders* (*DSM-III*) listed the condition as multiple personality disorder. In 1994, *DSM IV* changed that to the current name "dissociative personality disorders" and recognized three types; that term remains in *DSM-5* published in 2013.

It seems that everything about DID is controversial, including what causes it. The following two main ideas are presented as causes:

Reaction to trauma. The person faced a tremendous trauma in childhood, when the formation of the brain and personality are the most fragile. The trained therapist may trace the causal condition to disturbed and altered sleep, changes in environment, and severe trauma, which are usually extreme, repetitive physical, sexual, or emotional abuse. The personality is disassociated from the situation as a coping mechanism. The relationship between the abuse, detachment, and lack of social support may all point to DID.

Inappropriate psychotherapeutic techniques. The psychiatrist, in interviewing, may have encouraged the person to describe the symptoms of DID. This is a highly debated model; it is thought that the media plays a part in enhancing portrayals of DID.

WHAT ARE THE SIGNS AND SYMPTOMS OF DID?

In addition to the presence of two or more distinct personalities, other symptoms may include:

- Unhealthy mental thoughts, such as depression, suicide, and anxiety; the person may have attempted suicide
- Convinced that things around themselves are distorted and unreal
- Sense of detachment from self
- A blurred sense of identity (I am not me)
- An unusual amount of stress or problems that the person is not handling; these stressors can be in relationships, work, or other important areas of life

HOW IS IT DIAGNOSED?

People with DID may also have many comorbid disorders, such as schizophrenia bipolar disorder, epilepsy, borderline personality, and Asperger syndrome.

How to diagnose DID is one of the most controversial of all disorders, and results are disputed even among experts.

WHAT IS THE TREATMENT?

There is a lack of consensus regarding treatment. Common treatment methods include cognitive behavior therapy, insight-oriented therapies, hypnotherapy, and some medications. The International Society for the Study of Trauma and Dissociation has guidelines to assist therapists in treating individuals, but again, different practitioners disagree on interpretation of the guidelines.

A CELEBRITY WITH DID

Herschel visited the ramshackle school in Wrightsville, Georgia that he once attended, which brought up many memories, most of them bad. He was a very large, overweight boy who had no friends and was constantly picked on. He had a severe stuttering problem. He was always getting bullied and beat up—and he never fought back. He would even scrape up a few coins and give them to some students just so they would talk with him. Growing up in school was traumatic for him, and he now connects that trauma to the development of dissociative identity disorder.

Herschel's last name is Walker, and he is a football legend. He revealed his struggle with dissociative identity disorder in a book, *Breaking Free: My Life with Dissociative Identity Disorder*, in which he describes experiencing over a dozen alternate personalities, which nearly drove him to disaster.

Herschel Walker is probably one of the most impressive football players ever. In 1982, he became a household name among sports lovers when he gained recognition at the University of Georgia. He led the team to a national championship and was winner of the coveted Heisman trophy in 1982. He went on to play pro football and set records with the Dallas Cowboys and the Minnesota Vikings. He was later inducted into the Football Hall of Fame.

However, when he retired from football in 1997, he felt something that began to overwhelm him. He did not know that he was struggling with DID. He had several personalities, and it took him over 10 years to find out what his condition was. Some of his alters were the Hero, the Coach, the Enforcer, the Consoler, the Daredevil, and the Warrior. One time, the Warrior alter played Russian roulette with a gun held to his head. The other personas would never have done this; some of them were very good and compassionate. He had very sweet alters, and very violent ones. The disorder caused the breakup of his marriage and family.

Herschel states that he is much better now. He describes how therapy has helped him integrate all of the personalities. His goal in writing his book was to help people, and to let them know about this disorder.

For Further Information

Haddock, Deborah. *The Dissociative Identity Disorder Sourcebook*. New York: McGraw Hill, 2001.

Walker, H. *Breaking Free: My Life with Dissociative Identity Disorder*. New York: Simon and Schuster, 2008.

Erotomania: Obsessive Love

- Also known as Clérambault's syndrome
- A psychological condition in which a person has delusions that the object of his or her love feels the same love, but does not show it
- Usually the target of the affection is famous and glamorous
- Seen in persons with schizophrenia or bipolar disorders

On March 30, 1981, a young man named John Hinckley shot President Ronald Reagan in the chest as the president walked from the Hilton Hotel in Washington, DC to his car. Hinckley also seriously wounded several others. In a letter written to actress Jodie Foster, he revealed that he was doing this to impress her, and to let her know how much he loved her. He had sent her letters professing his love, in which he stated that it was their destiny to be together. He was found not guilty by way of insanity, and was committed to St. Elizabeth's Hospital in Washington, DC, diagnosed with erotomania.

This condition should not be confused with a simple crush, which usually disappears in a short period of time. The condition is a real psychotic disorder, and is listed as such in the *Diagnostic and Statistical Manual of Mental Disorders 5* (*DSM-5*). Although this illness is rare, it usually commands attention because of the unusual presentation and relation to high-profile people.

WHAT IS EROTOMANIA?

Erotomania is a condition in which a person has the delusion that another individual, usually a stranger or famous person, is in love with them. It is a psychosis that usually accompanies schizophrenia, bipolar disorder, or delusional disorder. The person may send letters, phone calls, gifts, or stalk the person of his or her affection. He or she may believe that the person is also in love with them, and is sending secretly coded messages.

In 1921 the French psychiatrist Gaetam de Clérambault (1872–1934) published a paper titled *Les psychoses passionelles*, in which he described how a delusional person thought a person of higher status was in love with him. Sometimes the disorder is called by Clérambault's name, at other times, erotomania. The word comes from two Greek roots: *eros,* meaning "love" and *mania,* meaning "madness for."

Finding the cause is not easy. The psychiatrist may only theorize. The most accepted cause is that it is somehow rooted in childhood with a lack of parental affection.

WHAT ARE THE SIGNS AND SYMPTOMS?

There are three main symptoms. The first is the delusion that the individual is madly in love with the other and is convinced that that person is secretly in love with him or her also. He or she is convinced that the person returns that love, and expresses it through special glances, signals, or mental messages. If the person is a celebrity, he or she is thought to be sending secret messages through the media. The individual may then stalk the person he or she loves. The individual may harass the other person by sending love letters, flowers, and making telephone calls.

HOW IS IT DIAGNOSED?

Erotomania is a real psychosis. There are several presentations of the disorder, with the major one being a belief that another person is secretly in love with them. According to *DSM-5*, the person should show the delusional behavior for at least a month. The object of the affection is usually a rock star, actor, or someone in a powerful position. The person believes that the love object communicates with him or her in subtle ways, such as body posture, glances, smiles, or other ways. Sometimes, a political figure may be thought to be sending messages to them through media such as radio or television. The individual may then stalk the person and become violent to anyone who might stand in the way. People with the disorder are completely unaware of the psychiatric implications.

WHAT IS THE TREATMENT?

Again, treatment is not simple. Finding the root of the problem can be elusive. Because the condition may be associated with other psychotic problems, these will have to be diagnosed and treated also. The use of antipsychotic drugs may reduce the symptoms of delusion.

However, the prognosis is not good. For example, even after years of treatment and incarceration in the hospital, John Hinckley still obsesses about Jodie Foster. Pictures have been found in his room that said, "Napoleon and Josephine; John and Jodie."

For Further Information

Orion, Doreen R. *I Know You Really Love Me: A Psychiatrist's Journal of Erotomania, Stalking, and Obsessive Love.* New York: Macmillan, 1997.

Folie à Deux: Shared Psychotic Beliefs

- Also known as: shared psychotic disorder; induced delusional disorder; Laségue-Falret Syndrome; infectious insanity
- Two or more people share the same delusional beliefs
- A primary inducer transmits the delusion to a secondary person or persons
- Treatment can be extremely difficult

Mrs. L. was a poet, but her submissions were always returned "rejected." She was convinced that the rejections of her poetry were because the establishment was against her, and told everyone of her problems with publishers. She even convinced Joe, her husband, that there was a conspiracy in the literary world to keep her from publishing. He became a true believer that the conspiracy existed, and even engaged his children in the belief. According to the psychiatrist handling the case, Mrs. L. was diagnosed with schizophrenia, and Joe and the children with induced psychosis. Mrs. L. was treated with antipsychotic drugs, but when evaluated six years later, she and Joe still held the belief that she was being persecuted by the establishment. The children moved to other places, and did not share the belief. Mrs. L. and Joe had folie à deux.

WHAT IS FOLIE À DEUX?

Folie à deux is a psychotic condition in which a delusional belief is transferred to another person or persons. The French term literally means "psychosis by two." However, it can be transmitted to three or more, or even to the masses.

History is filled with tragic stories of mass delusions. On October 1938, millions of Americans panicked as they thought Martians were invading, the result of a broadcast of H. G. Wells's story *War of the Worlds*. In November 1978, Reverend Jim Jones, a leader of the People's Temple, convinced 909 followers to drink Kool Aid laced with cyanide at Jonestown, Guyana. These people were convinced of conspiracies against their group, and that impending doom was upon them. People become part of groupthink or mass hysteria; the thinking of the group is contagious.

In 1877, two French psychiatrists Charles Laségue (1816–1883) and Jean Pierre Falret (1794–1870) first detailed this phenomenon. They called it infectious insanity, and described how one with a delusional disorder could induce others to follow his or her beliefs. The condition is listed in *Diagnostic and Statistical Manual of Mental Disorders* (*DSM*), which lays out the conditions for diagnoses. *DSM* states that it cannot be diagnosed if the delusion is ordinarily accepted in the person's culture.

No one knows the exact cause. The people involved are quite adept at hiding the delusion, and telling health care professionals what they want to hear. Many of the cases involved have come from families. Researchers have shown that sisters with folie à deux exceed all other combinations. Other combinations are husband and wife, and mother and child pairs.

One of the group tends to be the inducer or dominant personality. That person is usually more intelligent, stubborn, and overbearing. The submissive one is usually less intelligent and has considerable self-esteem issues. People living in isolation from society may have unhealthy relationships that develop into shared delusions. In one case, 72-year-old Ed and his 79-year-old sister Sue had major issues with their neighbors. Sue, the dominant personality, was convinced their neighbors intended to harm them, and had made up bizarre stories that the couple was having sex with their animals. The neighbors complained to police, who finally had the siblings committed for mental evaluation. They were treated with antipsychotic medicine, which they did not take after they returned home, and the delusions continued until their deaths.

The bizarre nature of the condition makes it fodder for stories and film. A 2006 film called *Bug* tells of Agnes, a waitress in Oklahoma, who meets Peter, a recently discharged soldier. He convinces her that when he was in the military, he was the subject of biological experiments by the government, and that they are both now being infected with microscopic bugs.

WHAT ARE THE SIGNS AND SYMPTOMS?

There are some subtypes of folie à deux: folie imposée and folie simultanée. Folie imposée sounds very much like the English word "impose." In this type, a dominant person, known as the primary, inducer, or principal, has a delusional belief related to some type of psychosis. The ideas are shared and pushed on a second party, called the acceptor or associate. Left to his or her own devices, the secondary may not have the delusion. An example would be that one of a pair of lovers is convinced that their only way out is to commit suicide together. The primary person, usually the male, convinces the female that this is the only way to go—and they would go out together. This nearness of death gives them energy and purpose. Survivors of suicide describe how the attempt suddenly gave their life meaning again. Planning the suicide was thrilling and exciting, and gave them release from the misery they had experienced.

The second type occurs when two people who have the psychosis influence each other in the delusions. The interaction of the two means that one feeds upon the other, and further promotes the delusions.

HOW IS IT DIAGNOSED?

This condition is diagnosed according to the descriptions in *DSM-5* of criteria for people with shared psychotic disorder. In Europe, is it diagnosed in ICD-10 diagnostic criteria as an induced delusional disorder.

WHAT IS THE TREATMENT?

Obviously, the treatment is very difficult, because many people can hide the real delusions. Even when they are committed to a facility and take medications, the delusions persist. Sometimes if the secondary person is separated from the primary, he or she can be treated with some success.

For Further Information

Enoch, D. and H. Ball. "Folie à deux (et Folie à plusieurs)." In D. Enoch, and H. Ball. *Uncommon psychiatric syndromes*, 4th ed. London: Arnold, 2001.

Wehmeier, P. M., N. Barth, and H. Remschmidt. "Induced Delusional Disorder: A Review of the Concept and an Unusual Case of Folie à Famille." *Psychopathology* 36 (1): 37–45, 2003.

Hybristophilia: Loving Men Behind Bars

- Mostly women who fall in love with men behind bars who have committed heinous crimes
- A type of paraphilia
- Both active and passive forms of the condition
- Reasons for such behavior can vary

In 2003, Dagmar Polzin, a German waitress was waiting at a bus stop in Hamburg when she saw a poster campaigning against the death penalty, with a picture of Bobby Lee Harris. Harris was on death row for the brutal stabbing of his boss during a robbery on a shrimp boat. She was overwhelmed by the picture, began writing to him, and within a year, she and Harris were engaged. She moved to America to live with his family, who lived near the prison. What makes women like Dagmar fall in love with someone who has committed a crime, and go to such lengths to be with him, appears to most people as puzzling. Dagmar has a condition called hybristophilia—women who fall in love with men behind bars, many of whom have committed heinous acts. Psychologists tell us that these prison romances are in no danger of dying out.

WHAT IS HYBRISTOPHILIA?

Hybristophilia is a condition in which a person is physically aroused and attracted to people who are incarcerated for heinous crimes. The person might have committed rape, murder, torture, and be a serial killer. More women than men appear to have this attraction, and the women are not just those who are in the lower socio-economic groups. They may be teachers, lawyers, or other professionals, and come from all segments of society. For example, Carlos the Jackal, a British serial killer, became engaged to his attorney. A Scottish criminal, Jimmy Boyle, married a psychiatrist whom he met in prison.

Hybristophilia is a form of paraphilia, or abnormal sexual drives. There are about 495 forms of paraphilia listed in the *Diagnostic and Statistical Manual of Mental Disorders 5*. These types range from those who derive sexual gratification from animals, called bestiality, to those who crave inanimate objects. Pedophilia, those who prey on children, is also one of the forms of paraphilia. Hybristophilia comes from the Greek roots *hubrizein*, meaning "to commit an outrage against someone," and *philia*, meaning "to like" or "to have a strong preference for." According to the definition, people with hybristophilia have a strong preference for those who are outside the law and have committed an outrageous act against society.

The reasons why these women may fall for such individuals is baffling. Psychologists and psychiatrists have many ideas; however, none of them have really been studied scientifically for causation. Following are some of the possible explanations that have been proposed:

- **Sense of glamour.** The relationship reinforces a sense of glamour about such individuals and their value system. Ted Bundy was an extremely good looking and charming man, whose appearance fit in with upper middle class values and ideals. The fact that he used his good looks and charm to lure his victims excites these women. During his trial, the courtroom was packed with suitors. He received hundreds of love letters while he was incarcerated. During the trial, he proposed to Carole Anne Boone in the courtroom, while he was on the stand, then married her. She had a daughter by him, but later got a divorce, changed her name, and disappeared.
- **Fame and notoriety may increase their social standing and the amount of attention they receive.** In November 2013, a 25-year-old woman named Star, in an interview with *Rolling Stone* magazine and CNN, declared her intention to marry 79-year-old Charles Manson. Whether the marriage ever takes place or not, she is getting attention that she never had previously. Manson, known for his charisma and charm, gets more fan mail than any other serial killer. The women may also get a book or movie deal.
- **A relationship with a person behind bars gives the other person control over the relationship.** According to Sheila Isenberg, author of *Women Who Love Men Who Kill*, many of the women themselves have been in abusive or violent relationships. The men are behind bars, making the women completely in charge of the relationship. Most of them communicate only through letters or for a few hours on visiting days. They do not have to cook for him or do

laundry. They fanaticize about what it would be like if the man was not in jail, knowing full well that he is.

- **Religious reasons.** Evangelical fervor is an obvious motivator. Some of the women hope that they can change or convert the man, and that really he is a sweet little boy who was just the victim of circumstances. Being intelligent and great manipulators, the prisoners can easily encourage these people.
- **Agreeing with extreme ideology.** Terrorists Anders Breivik and Dzhokhar Tsarnaev have received many letters agreeing with their actions and expressing admiration. One man who was placed on death row for murdering his entire family was sent a letter by a woman who admired his courage and said she wanted to do the same to her family. When Scott Peterson was convicted of murdering his wife, he immediately got sympathy letters from women.

WHAT ARE THE SIGNS AND SYMPTOMS?

Two types of people with hybristophilia exist: passive and aggressive. Although each type has its distinct characteristics, both types end up in abusive and unhealthy relationships.

- **Passive hybristophilia.** These individuals are the letter writers who send "fan mail" to the men in prison. Known as serial killer groupies (SKGs), they write letters to men behind bars, but usually have no interest in taking part in their criminal activity. They will find reasons and excuses for the behavior of the men, and believe that these men would never harm them. Many have rescue fantasies and believe they can change the person. These women are easily manipulated by the people they fall for.
- **Aggressive hybristophilia.** These women desire to be part of the criminal agenda, and will help their lovers in any criminal way. They never accept the fact that these men are psychopaths, and are capable of manipulating them.

The women must find ways to make connections with the men behind bars. It takes a lot of effort to get into the prison system and make contact with the person who is the object of her desire. Some of them will volunteer at the prison in order to meet the men. Many of the women will try to contact several men before they find a suitable match.

WHAT IS THE CAUSE?

Psychologists have only theories for the cause of this condition. Some believe that the women are submissive victims and others think that the women are narcissistic, wanting attention. Some may have wanted to get a published book out of it.

HOW IS IT DIAGNOSED?

The women who are in these situations would probably not admit that they have a problem, and would not submit themselves to therapy.

WHAT IS THE TREATMENT?

Most of the women make a conscious choice and extreme effort to cultivate the relationship, and have no desire to be treated; however, if they are detected as dangerous to the community, the court may order some type of behavior intervention. There are many types of treatment: psychotherapy, cognitive behavior therapy, group therapy, hypnosis, and medications such as antidepressants or mood stabilizers.

For Further Information
Parker, R. J. *Serial Killer Groupies*. Toronto: R. J. Parker Publishing, 2014.

Hypomania: Mania with Creative Energy

- A feature of bipolar II
- Person displays a mood that is energetic, talkative, and creative
- May appear as a positive trait
- Many people with bipolar II are highly functional

Roberta was from an old and respected family in the city. As a teenager, she was recognized as a debutante. She completed her master's degree and was a popular teacher at the community college. But all was not well with Roberta. She had occasions in which her behavior was erratic and differed from the norm. At times she was overly talkative and would seek out strangers in a group; at other times, she was just a shy person. There were times when she was extremely creative; then she would quickly lose interest in the projects she was promoting. Her personal life was chaotic with several failed marriages. She lived alone in a large beautiful house.

She retired early from her teaching but was still pleasant to those who met her. One night the community was shocked: she had been smoking in bed, and had set the house on fire. Roberta died of smoke inhalation before firefighters could save her. Roberta's behavior was typical of a condition called hypomania. It was revealed to friends after her death that she had hypomania.

WHAT IS HYPOMANIA?

Hypomania is a less severe form of mania. Bipolar mania, depression, and hypomania are all symptoms of bipolar disorder. Hypomania is a feature of bipolar II and cyclothymia, the mood swings between depression and elevated feelings. People with hypomania have a less severe form of mania. Some physicians do not consider it a problem, because the person can function very well, feel good, and be quite productive. However, for people with bipolar disorder, this can evolve into mania or switch to serious depression.

The word "hypomania" comes from the Greek: *hypo* meaning "under" and *mania* literally meaning "madness." When psychiatry first emerged in the 19th century, mania had the meaning of craziness or insanity. However, the term has evolved today to mean a sense of euphoria or excitability. Later, it was noted that some people do not have the same issues as those with true bipolar depression, and there should be some condition that was not quite as severe.

German psychiatrist Emanuel Ernst Mendel (1839–1907) in 1881 recommended that hypomania be used to describe a condition that was less severe that than of true bipolar disorder. Later, in the 20th century, a narrower definition of hypomania evolved. Now the hypomanic episode is not a disorder itself, but a part of a type of bipolar disorder II. There are two distinct differences: the problem is not serious enough to cause problems with the person working or socializing with others; psychotic features are not present.

The primary difference is the absence of psychotic symptoms. Although they may have some grandiose ideas, it is not as exaggerated as those with bipolar disorder. Also, the person can function well in everyday life, which is quite different from those with bipolar depression. Some people may have hypersexuality and interest in lewd and lascivious activities. The creative aspect of the person with hypomania is a hallmark. That individual may have a flood of ideas that flow with boundless energy. The person may be unusually driven to succeed.

The condition may be caused by several things. One of the most common is taking certain medications, which were prescribed to treat other conditions. Eliminating those drugs may treat the condition.

WHAT ARE THE SIGNS AND SYMPTOMS?

As listed in *DSM-5*, the person should have 3 or more of the following symptoms to a significant degree:

- The person must have an inflated sense of self-esteem or a feeling of grandiosity.
- The person may not have a need for sleep. He may get along with only three or four hours, and feel rested and functional with minimum rest.

- The individual is more talkative and outgoing at times that is different from her usual personality trait.
- She may talk rapidly and have ideas that are seemingly free flowing and sometimes unrelated to the subject; it is obvious that the mind is racing from one idea to another.
- The person is easily distracted. He may be thinking along one track and then suddenly change to another completely different one.
- There may be an increase in goal-related actives, such an increased sociability either at work or school,
- The person may do activities that are dangerous or threatening or that have negative consequences, such as foolish business investments, buying sprees, or sexual indiscretions.

For someone with bipolar disorder II, the disorder can go into mania or can switch into serious depression. The person also can develop false ideas and may stand very strongly for their ideas, and cannot be swayed from them even when they are shown to be in error. Because they think they have superhuman powers, they may consider themselves to god-like.

HOW IS IT DIAGNOSED?

This condition is listed in the current *Diagnostic and Statistical Manual of Mental Disorders* (*DSM-5*) as an area related to bipolar II. Although it is not as severe as other illnesses, it is recognized because it can be so disruptive to one's life.

WHAT IS THE TREATMENT?

Medications such as mood stabilizers that include valproic acid and lithium carbonate may be used.

For Further Information

Doran, Christopher M. *The Hypomania Handbook: The Challenge of Elevated Mood*. Philadelphia: LWW, 2007.

Jerusalem Syndrome: A Visit to the Holy City

- A state of intense delusion brought on by a visit to the Holy Land
- Can affect Jews, Christians, and Muslims

- Affected individuals adopt "biblical behavior"
- 470 tourists were treated in a mental facility between 1979 and 1993

Jerusalem is considered the holy city to the world's three major religions: Christianity, Islam, and Judaism. It hosts over one and a half million visitors each year. Many of the visitors attach a great significance to the city, and come away with good feelings. Jews find the Wailing Wall and sites of the temple meaningful; Christians are uplifted when following Jesus of Nazareth's last steps or visiting the site of the open tomb. However, some tourists do not just come and go. They develop a psychosis known as Jerusalem syndrome.

WHAT IS JERUSALEM SYNDROME?

Jerusalem syndrome is a psychological reaction to visiting the city of Jerusalem. It can manifest in Jews, Muslims, and Christians of many different backgrounds. In the 1930s, Israeli psychiatrist Dr. Heinz Herman, a founder of psychiatric research in Israel, first described the disorder. The syndrome may have been noted in other religious places such as Mecca and Rome, and other cases have been described as occurring in Jerusalem during the 19th century.

However, it was Dr. Yair Bar-El, former director of Kfar Shaul Mental Health Center in Jerusalem, who researched 470 tourists who had been declared temporarily insane. He has estimated that about 20 people a year are affected. According to Bar-El, 66 percent were Jews, 33 percent were Christians of various denominations, and 1 percent had no known religious affiliation. The occurrences were mostly in the summer months and during holiday seasons. However, as the year 2000 approached and tourists were anticipating the apocalypse, the number bloomed to about 50 cases a week, instead of 20 per year.

The first glimpse of the dramatic setting of Israel and the shock of actually seeing it may affect some visitors. Most of the people fit into the type 3—those who have no previous history of mental illness. Ages of the people ranged from 18 to 70, with a median age of 35. Many of them had attended higher education, and were not necessarily connected to a religious institution.

Jerusalem syndrome may be similar to other disorders that occur when one comes into contact with a place of great history. A similar disorder is called Stendhal syndrome, in which one has a similar reaction to great works of art.

WHAT ARE THE SIGNS AND SYMPTOMS?

People with this syndrome are thought to demonstrate proper behavior before coming to Jerusalem. When they see and hear about the holy sites, their behavior changes. They may adopt a role that they perceive is "biblical behavior." They travel through the streets singing psalms or praise songs, being Bible characters such as Moses, John the Baptist or Christ, and wearing a sheet from the hotel.

Some researchers have claimed that the people were mentally unstable before they came. However, Bar-El divided them into three groups: (1) visitors who were mentally ill when leaving their country of origin, who simply imposed Jerusalem syndrome on a previous psychotic illness; (2) people who were not ill but had deeply ingrained ideas that were exacerbated by the visit; And (3) sane people, who were business people, teachers, or other professionals, with no previous mental illness, but who had had a "brief psychotic episode." Their symptoms may include anxiety, agitation, and nervousness. They may have a desire to split away from the group and spend lots of time cleansing themselves. They may shout Bible verses or march to a holy place such as the Wailing Wall. They may deliver sermons that are obviously not prepared and sound disjointed.

Most of the time, people with the syndrome cause no problems. However, in 1969 an Australian tourist with Jerusalem syndrome set fire to the Al-Aqsa Mosque, the third holiest site in Sunni Islam. Tensions that were already strained in that part of the world erupted in citywide riots. Since that time, Israelis seek to treat all cases.

HOW IS IT DIAGNOSED?

The obvious change in behavior is a signal that something is awry. Israeli doctors know the condition and can diagnose it fairly quickly.

WHAT IS THE TREATMENT?

Currently, there is no treatment; however researchers are hoping for an effective diagnosis and treatment. Dr. Gregory Katz, a Russian psychiatrist, says that some of the patients are experiencing jet lag, and can be treated with melatonin or tranquilizers. If there is previous mental illness, the person may get antipsychotic drugs. Kfar Shaul Hospital can treat tourists in many languages.

For Further Information

Kalian, M., and E. Witztum. "Facing a Holy Space: Psychiatric Hospitalization of Tourists in Jerusalem." In *Sacred Space: Shrine, City, Land*, edited by Z. B. Kedar and R. J. Werblowsky. New York: NYU Press, 1998.

Kleptomania: A Need to Steal

- Prevalence: 0.6 percent of the general population
- More common among women than men
- Individuals feel a compulsive urge to steal

- 65 percent correlation in patients with bulimia, and 7 percent connection with those who have obsessive-compulsive disorders

Mary was the wife of an outstanding pillar of the church, and her father was a respected pastor. She lived an ideal life as a wife of a prosperous rancher, who provided her with everything that she wanted, and four delightful children. But Mary had a problem. She stole money from handbags that were left around the church or from petty funds from church dinners. Her husband knew that "she stole," but managed to cover it up whenever possible. Suddenly, for some mysterious reason, Mary forsook her home and family and went to live in a homeless community. The fact that she was a kleptomaniac was never talked about. Kleptomania is a condition that most people have heard about, but know little about.

WHAT IS KLEPTOMANIA?

Kleptomania is a complex disorder in which the person has an uncontrollable urge to steal. The items usually have no value to the person. Kleptomania is not shoplifting, which occurs when a person plans to pick up things that will be of value, to use for economic gain. The disorder is listed in the *Diagnostic and Statistical Manual of Mental Disorders 5*.

People with kleptomania, sometimes called "kleptos," steal for the thrill. Some persons report that during the act there is an altered state of consciousness that is considered depersonalization. They may act in a dream-like state. Before the act, the person may report a tension or urge that is released once the object is stolen. Guilt always occurs afterwards. Obviously, this behavior leads to personal distress, problems with the law, marital stress, and personal dysfunction. Many of the thefts are in plain view of law enforcement officials.

The condition was first described in 1816 and classified as an impulse control disorder. In the past, because most of the people with kleptomania were female, doctors proposed that it was related to a female condition that they called "hysteria." "Hysteria" comes from the Greek word *hyster,* meaning "uterus." An entire group of disorders, especially those with great emotional impact, were considered to be related to the female reproductive organs. This belief was held throughout the 19th century and continued into the early 20th century. These beliefs subsided in the second part of the 20th century.

WHAT ARE THE SIGNS AND SYMPTOMS?

Five major features of kleptomania follow:

1. The person has a failure to resist stealing the unneeded object. Unlike a shoplifter, he or she does not go into the store with the intent to steal anything. Many of the things they steal have absolutely no value.

2. Before committing the theft, there is a tremendous amount of tension. The tension is part of the compulsion.
3. After and during the theft, the experience is gratifying and very pleasurable.
4. The theft does not stem from antagonism or revenge, and is not a part of a fantasy.
5. The theft is not related to the person having a behavior disorder, manic episode, or antisocial personality disorder. The guilt afterwards may cause them to return the objects to the store.

These symptoms suggest an obsessive-compulsive type of disorder. Other similar personality disorders may include mood swings, eating disorders such as bulimia, anxiety disorders, and drug use. Some researchers think there may be a genetic component, because close relatives may have a substance abuse disorder or obsessive compulsive disorder.

HOW IS IT DIAGNOSED?

How to diagnose the disorder continues to be a debatable topic among psychiatrists. According to the *Diagnostic and Statistical Manual of Mental Disorders (DSM-5)*, the following characteristics are the diagnostic criteria for kleptomania:

- An urge to steal things that are not essential for private use or for economic value
- Escalating sense of pressure before the theft
- Satisfaction and fulfillment after the theft
- No revenge or antagonism exists; the theft is not a behavior disorder, manic episode, or antisocial personality disorder

WHAT IS THE TREATMENT?

Treatment of the condition is fairly difficult, because it is so poorly understood and often undetected. Family members may recognize the problem but aid in the cover up.

When the disorder is detected by extensive psychological and physical interviews, the treatment may be multifaceted. One of the first things is to determine whether the person has other mental disorders. Once there is a determination, the psychiatrist will work on creating impulse control. The person will be taught to look carefully at the triggers of the impulse. The following two psychological strategies may be used:

- **Cognitive-behavior theory.** This psychotherapeutic approach uses a combination of behavioral therapy and cognitive therapy to help the person understand the problem. The person will then develop goals to help him or her overcome the problem and assess those goals often. The person can reward him or herself when consistently reaching the goals.

- **Rational emotive therapy.** The psychiatrist helps the person focus on uncovering irrational beliefs that have led to negative emotions. The person wants to be happy, but these impulses will not lead to that goal. The person must replace these negative feelings with reasonable alternatives.
- **Drug treatment.** Some people have responded to selective serotonin reuptake inhibitors (SSRIs), a form of antidepressant. Others have found that opioid antagonists and mood stabilizers may help. Some other medications have been suggested.

One of the problems with kleptomania is that not much is known about the disorder. Very few controlled studies have been done with either psychological or medical interventions. In addition, there is little information about prevention, except for general strategies such as having a positive and healthy upbringing that will reduce stress.

For Further Information

Goldman, Marcus J. *Kleptomania: The Compulsion to Steal: What Can Be Done?* Far Hills, NJ: New Horizon Press, 1997.

Micropsia and Macropsia: Alice in Wonderland Syndrome

- Rare perceptual disorder
- Body size and objects appear larger or smaller than they actually are
- Numerous possible causes, including viral infections, seizures, drug use, or migraines
- No specific treatment

In 1865 Reverend Charles Lutwidge Dodgson, aka Lewis Carroll (1832–1898), penned a story about a little girl named Alice who became bored just sitting by a stream and looking at nature. She saw an unusual, fully clothed white rabbit and followed it into its hole. She fell a long way and landed in an attractive garden. She was hungry, and saw a cake and a bottle with a label that read "DRINK ME." She drank from the bottle, and immediately began to grow until she was so tall she hit her head against the ceiling. The objects, animals, and people all appeared small to her. From this story, the name Alice in Wonderland was given to a special syndrome in which objects appear out of proportion to the individual.

WHAT IS MICROPSIA AND MACROPSIA?

Alice in Wonderland syndrome (AIWS) or micropsia/macropsia is a psychopathological condition in which time, space, and body image are distorted. The person may feel that the whole body or body parts have changed. Objects appear to be different from what they are. The most common distortion is micropsia, in which things appear smaller than they actually are. The word origins are from the Greek: *micro*, meaning "small" and *macro* meaning "large." Combined with the root *opt*, meaning "to see," the condition describes either a small or a large world. Someone has described micropsia as looking backwards through binoculars. Although several diseases or disorders may have these distorted visuals, it is generally considered to be an area related to brain processing, and not some malfunction of the eye.

In 1952 C. W. Lippman in the *Canadian Medical Journal* first described the condition, but the name "Alice in Wonderland Syndrome" was given in an article written by John Todd (1914–1987), an English psychiatrist, in 1955. Sometimes the condition is referred to as the Cheshire Cat syndrome, another character from Alice in Wonderland. In 1968, the British physician Eric George Lapthorne Bywaters (1910–2003) described how common it was for young children to experience the distortion of the body, but they usually outgrow that tendency. For adults who experience that feeling, it is truly like living in wonderland.

That individuals could see things that were so disparately disproportionate to their actual size has fascinated several literary giants. In addition to Carroll, another British writer, Jonathan Swift, wrote a famous novel *Gulliver's Travels,* in which Gulliver goes to an island inhabited by the Lilliputians, a group of very tiny people. That is an alternate name for this disorder.

Many clinical conditions may be related to AIWS. Following are some of the conditions that have been associated with the condition:

- **Epstein-Barr condition.** The Epstein-Barr virus is a herpes virus that causes infectious mononucleosis. The presence of visual distortions may be one of the first symptoms of this condition. The distortions are also a symptom of Epstein-Barr viral infection. Neurologist Sheen Aurora performed a functional magnetic resonance imaging (fMRI)exam of a girl when she was experiencing the distortions. (An fMRI takes an actual picture of an event as it is occurring.) She found that a burst of abnormal electrical energy slowed or shut off the normal blood flow to the vision area of the brain that distinguishes size, shape, and color. This virus may also cause swelling in the cornea, which will cause a dislocation of certain cells in the eye.
- **Seizures.** Micropsias occur most often in seizures, especially in a type called temporal epilepsy. Most of the auras that occur with seizures last only a few seconds to a few minutes.

- **Migraines.** Migraine headaches have an initial period of attack that begins with an aura, a time when the person feels the onset of the migraine. Micropsia is common during this stage. The symptom occurs about 30 minutes before the beginning of the migraine.
- **Drug use.** Certain kinds of hallucinogenic drugs can cause micropsia. The hallucinations may cause a flashback similar to that of LSD. Long-term use of cocaine may cause a chronic condition. A drug called zolpidem, used to treat insomnia, may cause micropsia as a side effect. Dextromethorphan, a common ingredient of cough syrup, may cause the symptoms, as well has certain prescription medicines such as oxycodone or hydrocodone.
- **Certain psychological problems.** Certain people may have such anxiety or other psychological issues that the condition may be a part of those issues.

WHAT ARE THE SIGNS AND SYMPTOMS?

The person with AIWS experiences visual illusions. These are distortions of form, size, and color; objects may be seen to be backwards. Generally, the components of the physiology of the eye are normal. The term "Lilliputian" is used to describe the symptom whereby an object appears smaller or larger than it actually is. Patients may experience either micropsia or macropsia. Most patients are aware that the perceptions are not reality. Dr. Fiorenzo Ceriani and his colleagues at the University of Milan found that many of his patients could actually imagine the sizes of objects and even calculate the differences between them.

The symptoms vary with each person. For example, one person reported seeing a car the size of a small poodle. Another saw their body parts shrink and then grow. Touch and space perception may happen. A patient described that the ground felt like a sponge under foot; another described going through a hallway that never ends.

HOW IS IT DIAGNOSED?

Because of the varied causes, diagnosis may be very difficult, and will vary among cases. Tests such as electroencephalogram (EEG) can check for medial temporal epilepsy. The Amsler grid test can be used to detect macular degeneration. However, epilepsy is a disturbance of perception rather than a physical condition itself, and is present with many these disorders.

WHAT IS THE TREATMENT?

Currently, no current treatment exists for AIWS, as it is not commonly known or understood. The biggest causes appear to be migraines, which can be treated with certain drug protocols and diet. However, AIWS is really untreatable, and may in time wear itself out.

For Further Information

"Alice in Wonderland syndrome." In *Taber's Cyclopedic Medical Dictionary*. Philadelphia: F. A. Davis Company, 2009.

Cinbis, M., and S. Aysun. "Alice in Wonderland Syndrome as an Initial Manifestation of Epstein-Barr Virus Infection." *British Journal of Ophthalmology* 76 (5): 316, 1992.

Munchausen Syndrome: Playing Sick

- Person pretends to be sick to get attention
- Munchausen syndrome by proxy is when a person hurts another person in their care, to get sympathy or attention
- May be related to serious illness or trauma in childhood
- Difficult to diagnose

In the 1993 *Guinness Book of Records*, William McIlhoy, a resident of the United Kingdom, showed how he was an expert at being sick. Over a period of 50 years, he had 400 operations in 100 different hospitals, using 22 different names. Britain's National Health Services paid out more than $4 million for his treatments. There was only one problem: he was not sick. McIlhoy had Munchausen syndrome; he pretended that he had physical or psychological illnesses to get attention and sympathy. After years of convincing doctors and hospital staff that he was sick and exaggerating his illnesses, he gave up and spent his remaining years in a retirement home.

WHAT IS MUNCHAUSEN SYNDROME?

Munchausen Syndrome occurs when people pretend they are sick, just to get attention. They may go from doctor to doctor to find answers, although they are not sick. Another form is called Munchausen syndrome by proxy (MSBP), in which an adult may hurt a child or another individual to get money, gifts, and attention from others.

The term "Munchausen syndrome" has a unique history. Baron Karl Friedrich Hieronymus Freiherr von Münchausen (1720–1797) was a Prussian nobleman who hired himself out as a mercenary to the Russian army. Münchausen traveled widely throughout Russia and Germany, telling unbelievable and exaggerated stories about his exploits and escapades. The tales were so wildly outrageous that people were fascinated. The writer Rudolph Erich Raspe collected his stories and published them as *The Surprising Adventures of Baron Munchausen*.

In 1951 Richard Asher (1912–1969), an eminent British endocrinologist, encountered some patients who told wild stories about what was happening to them. These individuals made up the stories and feigned illnesses. Asher had heard of Münchausen and his outrageous stories. The doctor then named the condition after the Baron, observing that both the Baron and the patients told unusual stories about themselves that were absolutely untrue. At first, the term described all made-up disorders, but now relates only to those who have the severest form of made-up disorders that affect the person's life. The term "factitious" is used to describe conditions that are feigned, contrived, or artificial.

There are two types of Munchausen syndrome. The first is the type in which a person, like McIlhoy, feigns illness to get sympathy and attention. The second type is called Munchausen syndrome by proxy (MSBP), in which a person makes up the fabrications of illness of someone in his or her care. The term "by proxy" means "through a substitute." Both of these factitious illnesses are serious mental illnesses, and associated with people who have severe emotional disorders.

Munchausen syndrome is not hypochondria, the condition of people who truly believe they are sick, when they really are not. The person with Munchausen knows he or she is not sick, and purposefully lies about the condition. Often, they have studied the condition and know a lot about it, so that they can fake it. Anyone on the outside may have difficulty telling the difference.

Those people with Munchausen may be a great danger to themselves and to others. They have been known to jump from moving cars, fall out of high windows, or do other dangerous things that will result in broken bones or damaged organs. Women have been known to get pregnant and then force a miscarriage or abortion in order to get sympathy. In addition, to keep others from finding out the truth, they may go as far as to commit murder to cover up the evidence. Another situation may occur, called "Munchausen by internet syndrome," in which people tell very sad stories to get donations from unsuspecting people.

Munchausen syndrome by proxy (MSBP) occurs when an adult presents a child as ill or injured to a doctor or a medical facility. The person may do it not for sympathy, but to get money. According to the American Professional Society on the Abuse of Children, this is considered a form of child abuse, and is prosecuted as a criminal act under the Child Abuse Prevention and Treatment Act of 1974. For example, John was 16 months old when his mother brought him to the clinic for vomiting, bleeding, diarrhea, seizures, and poor feeding. At the age of two months, he had been brought in for sleep apnea, and at six months, for seizures. When the physicians made a covert videotape, it showed the mother loving her child one minute and then trying to suffocate him the next. This mother is an example of a severe emotionally disturbed person. However, it may also be applied to adults who are in the care of someone with MSBP.

The person with Munchausen syndrome has serious psychological problems and perhaps has experienced childhood traumas or serious illness as a child. They have very low self-esteem. Many times they had aspirations of working as a doctor, or they might have a history of working in healthcare. It is more common among males, and in young or middle-aged adults.

WHAT ARE THE SIGNS AND SYMPTOMS?

The symptoms of both Munchausen syndrome and MSBP are similar. Both are very difficult to diagnose, and obviously the person will not seek medical help. Following are some of the symptoms displayed by people with Munchausen syndrome:

- The individual changes the story about symptoms or what happened to cause the illness.
- The person is sick all the time, with reoccurring illnesses that cannot be explained.
- The person may simulate or stimulate cardiac arrhythmias in order to gain medical attention. This is called arrhythmogenic Munchausen syndrome.
- The person will have lots of scars and many medical bills.
- They may say they are ill, then do things that a sick person would not do, such as party, travel, or enjoy life.
- They may be unwilling to share information about previous treatments.
- The person may resist treatment or therapy.

Following are the things that may lead health professionals to suspect MSBP:

- The child may have alleged allergies to a variety of foods or drugs.
- The child has reoccurring illnesses that cannot be explained.
- Episodes occur only at home and never at school; child may be absent often from school.
- The mother is overly attentive and may refuse to leave the child's bedside.
- The mother follows the medical staff around and is extremely helpful in care.
- Symptoms cease when the mother is separated from the child.
- The mother has a personality disorder and may herself have Munchausen syndrome.

MSBP occurs mostly in women, and is usually connected with turmoil in a marriage, or if the father is not involved in childcare.

HOW IS IT DIAGNOSED?

Diagnosis is extremely difficult, because the person must admit what they have done in order to correct the problem. The doctor must examine the person's complete history. A misdiagnosis can be extremely harmful, because the person may also have borderline personality disorder, bipolar, anxiety disorders, or cognitive problems.

WHAT IS THE TREATMENT?

First the person must admit to deception, and determine to correct the problem. In MSBP, the individual must be monitored at all times, and promise to keep the child with the same doctor. Even then, the prognosis is poor.

English physician David Southall used covert video to observe 33 mothers abusing their children. When confronted, one mother said that she thought that if she did something drastic enough, someone would see how badly she needed help.

For Further Information

Feldman, Marc D. *Playing Sick?: Untangling the Web of Munchausen Syndrome, Munchausen by Proxy, Malingering, and Factitious Disorder*. London: Routledge Press, 2004.

Orthorexia: When Eating Healthy Becomes Unhealthy

- More common in women than men.
- Person is obsessed with healthy eating and may adopt habits that are detrimental to health.
- Condition differs from anorexia, in that the person is not concerned about weight loss, but in eating only pure and healthy foods.
- Not officially recognized as an eating disorder by the *Diagnostic and Statistical Manual of Mental Disorders*

When Karen was in high school, she really appreciated her nutrition classes, and began to adhere closely to the food pyramid that the government recommended. She read studies about eating, and took seriously that she should avoid trans fats, foods with artificial flavors, and meat. After deciding to become a vegan, she adopted a program of eating only organic raw fruits and vegetables. She was obsessed with eating only pure foods, and managed her diet very carefully. She preferred to go hungry than eat anything that was not healthy. By age 27, she weighed 68 pounds, had anemia, and osteoporosis. Karen possibly had a condition called orthorexia.

Orthorexia is not listed in any edition of the *Diagnostic and Statistical Manual of Mental Disorders*, nor in the European manuals of disorders. However, the condition has received lots of attention in the popular press recently.

WHAT IS ORTHOREXIA?

Orthorexia is a proposed eating disorder in which the person is obsessed with eating only pure and healthy foods. He or she is not concerned about losing weight, but is fixated on eating proper foods that he or she perceives to be correct. It becomes an obsession or compulsion, and may be compared to obsessive compulsive disorder (OCD).

In 1997, Steven Bratman, a physician, coined the term "orthorexia nervosa" by combining the Greek roots *ortho*, meaning "straight" or "correct" and *orexia*, meaning "appetite." It is patterned after the eating disorder "anorexia," which means "without appetite." The difference between the two, is that a person with anorexia is overly concerned with weight and body image, and the person with orthorexia is concerned about eating only to improve health. Bratman himself has a history of dealing with the disorder, both when he lived in a commune in the 1970s and after medical school, as a practitioner of alternative medicine in California. He has written extensively about the disorder in his book *Health Food Junkies: Orthorexia: Overcoming the Obsession with Healthful Eating.*

At this point the person's eating has become like an obsessive-compulsive disorder; now it is not only a physical issue, but a mental one. The isolation from others then leads to depression and mood swings or anxiety. It is similar to anorexia nervosa, in that both achieve control of their lives by guarding food intake. It is different in that a person with anorexia is concerned about weight; the one with orthorexia is concerned about healthy intake of food.

WHAT ARE THE SIGNS AND SYMPTOMS?

The symptoms appear to progress from one stage to another. The person may start out by avoiding foods that relate to asthma, digestive problems, or anxiety. She begins to read extensively about various foods and does not necessarily seek medical advice. She hears that certain foods such as fat, sugar, or salt may be "bad" for her and determines to avoid anything that has anything in it that could have an adverse effect on her health. She then may increase herbal or other supplements or probiotics/macrobiotics. Food preparation and selection becomes an obsession. She now avoids foods that have artificial colors, flavors, or preservatives, those treated with pesticides, or that have genetic modifications.

Next comes social isolation. Her obsession with food affects her life and her relationships with others. She may avoid others because she considers that she has power now, and that others who indulge in improper and unhealthy foods are weak. She does not want to eat out or dine at the homes of others, because they do not follow her strict standards of preparing food. Her feelings of self-esteem are tied to the obsession with food.

HOW IS IT DIAGNOSED?

Bratman has developed a 10-point questionnaire that includes such questions as: Are you spending more than three hours a day thinking about healthy food? Has the quality of your life decreased as the quality of your diet increased?

WHAT IS THE TREATMENT?

Nutritionists and medical professionals who recognize this disorder state that it is very difficult to treat. Those people who have been so convinced that what they are doing is good for them, may only realize a problem exists when they develop some real nutritional deficiency, such as anemia or osteoporosis, that affects their overall health. Because change addresses habits acquired over a number of years, it cannot be treated in just one session, but may take several sessions over a number of months.

For Further Information

Bratman, Steven. *Health Food Junkies: Orthorexia Nervosa—The Health Food Eating Disorder*. Easton, PA: Harmony, 2004.

Reel, Justine J. *Eating Disorders: An Encyclopedia of Causes, Treatment, and Prevention*. Santa Barbara, CA: ABC-CLIO, 2013.

Pica: Eating the Inedible

- May affect 10-30 percent of children ages one to six; much rarer among adults
- Person eats items that are not part of a normal diet
- May be caused by a number of factors, including developmental disabilities, psychological problems, neglect, and nutritional deficiencies
- Can cause serious health problems

Charles Domery (c. 1778 – after 1800), a mercenary in the Prussian Army, was always hungry and would eat anything. He was said to have eaten 174 cats in a year and devoured four to five pounds of grass each day. Serving on a ship, he began eating the severed leg of a sailor who had been hit by cannon fire, until his shipmates stopped him. He was captured by the British and put in prison. There he ate the prison cat, 20 rats that came into his cell, and all the prison candles. To say the least, he had an extreme case of a condition known as pica.

Pica is described in the *Diagnostic and Statistical Manual of Mental Disorders 5* (*DSM-5*) as a mental illness, although some experts relate it to nutritional needs and culture.

WHAT IS PICA?

Pica (pronounced PY-kah) is a condition in which a person eats items not considered part of a normal diet, such as ice, clay, chalk, sand, or dirt. At some point, young children put nonfood objects into their mouths or eat sand or dirt. However, people with pica have a pattern of eating items that have no nutritive value. They may even crave these items. The condition is listed in *DSM-IV* as common in people with developmental disabilities, such as autism, cognitive disability, and brain injury. However, there are some variations that may arise from cultural traditions, a deficiency such as iron imbalance, or even just many of the stressors of life.

In order to qualify for pica, the person must have the pattern of eating items that are not part of a normal diet for at least one month. The list of nonfood items that the person may crave is quite long. Following are some of the things that people with pica crave, notated first in their scientific names from *DSM*, followed by the explanation of the disorder:

- Geophagia - The person eats soil, clay, or chalk; a subset of this is lithophagia, when the person craves pebbles or rocks
- Pagophagia - The person is obsessed with eating ice or frost from a freezer
- Coprophagia - The person eats feces, usually animal, though it could be human feces
- Hyalophagia - The person craves glass
- Trichophagia - The person eats hair or wool
- Xylophagia - The person consumes wood or paper

Other items may include paint chips or plaster, corn or laundry starch, cigarette butts or ashes, mucus, urine, burnt match heads, buttons, toothpaste, coffee grounds, and soap.

Some eating patterns are related to culture. Among the African slaves in the United States in the 1800s, eating clay was very popular, as it was believed to supplement an iron-deficient diet. Even now, in some cultures, eating behaviors may be part of religious ceremonies. There is a tradition called Odowa, in which soft stones are eaten by pregnant women in Kenya.

A 13th-century Latin text first referenced pica as a disorder. The name "pica" comes from the Latin word for *magpie*. The magpie is a large black and white bird of the crow family, whose genus name is Pica. The magpie has very unusual eating behaviors and is known to eat just about anything. The condition was first mentioned in medical texts in 1563. Research on eating disorders over four centuries, from the 16th to the 20th centuries, mentioned pica as a symptom rather than a separate eating disorder. It was catalogued as a separate disorder in *DSM III* (1986 edition).

Pica is still one of the mysteries of eating disorders. Following are some of the situations that might be related to the cause:

- **Developmental disorders.** The person may have some type of developmental disability, such as autism, intellectual disability, or brain trauma.
- **Mental conditions.** The person may combine this disorder with an obsessive-compulsive disorder (OCD) and schizophrenia.
- **Pregnancy.** Pica occurring during pregnancy may be related to cravings. However, those who had pica as children or a family history of pica may be more at risk.
- **Nutritional deficiencies.** Some experts have speculated that a deficiency of iron or zinc may trigger certain cravings for things like clay or dirt. However, it has been shown that these substances do not supply the body with minerals.
- **Dieting.** People who are on diets may eat certain substances to give them a feeling of being full and avert hunger pangs.
- **Neglect or inadequate food.** Children who are left alone with no supervision, or who have not been fed, may eat nonfood items to assuage hunger.
- **Cultural practices.** Some religions or cultures may practice eating certain non-food items. People in some cultures believe that eating dirt will infuse magical spirits into their bodies.

WHAT ARE THE SIGNS AND SYMPTOMS?

There are three basic warning signs of pica:

1. The child must exhibit the pattern for at least one month or longer.
2. The nonfood item must be inappropriate for the child's developmental stage, such as older than 18 to 24 months.
3. The behavior is not part of a religious, ethnic, or cultural practice.

Most of the items that people with pica ingest are quite dangerous. Even the suspicion that pica may be present must lead to a medical assessment for many complications. Such conditions could be anemia, intestinal blockages from eating indigestible items such as hair, buttons or glass, poisons from lead or soap, or parasites from dirt or feces.

HOW IS IT DIAGNOSED?

If pica is suspected, a medical evaluation is important to assess anemia, intestinal blockages, or danger from other ingested items. The doctor will use blood tests and X-rays, as well as tests for possible infections. Other issues are probably present. Mental retardation, developmental disorders, or OCD must enter into consideration.

CASE HISTORY: THE LADY WHO ATE SEVEN SOFAS

Adele is a 31-year-old living in Bradenton, Florida. She recently went to a clinic for medical help for an unusual addiction. She has been eating sofas for 21 years. Her favorite snack is unzipping the covers of the pillows and munching down on the foam inside. Her snacking may occur as often as 15 times a day, and she eats probably the equivalent of a throw pillow a week. She has been eating foam since she was 10 years old.

This mother of five knows that the habit will soon kill her, but she simply cannot stop. About three years ago she woke up in the night with a terrible pain. When she arrived at the hospital, the doctors found a foam blockage about the size of a grapefruit in her lower intestine.

Doctors at the Digestive Health Center in Sarasota diagnosed her with pica, then were shocked when she told them she had another addiction—that of eating dirt. She has moved in with her sister, and took enough pillow cushions with her to do for a while. She is scheduled to enter a therapy center in California for people with strange addictions, and now believes it is time to get serious about quitting.

WHAT IS THE TREATMENT?

Treating pica can be difficult. Depending on the materials eaten and the effect, the medical team must work in close collaboration with a mental health team to keep the behavior from happening again. Pica that begins in childhood may last only a few months. Medication and behavioral therapy may be used if the person does not improve within a reasonable amount of time. However, the child with developmental disabilities may be more difficult to treat.

Nemours/Alfred I. duPont Hospital for Children recommends three things to prevent pica:

- Teach the child what is safe to eat
- Store craved items in a locked cabinet or out of reach
- Make sure the child gets a well-balanced diet

For Further Information

Connor, Jane. *Pica Eating – Overcoming Pica Eating Disorder for Life.* Printed by Amazon Digital Services, Inc., 2013.

Renfield Syndrome: Consuming Blood

- Person has an obsession with drinking blood
- Not recognized in either U.S. or European clinical manuals as a separate disorder
- Mostly affects males
- Afflicted individuals may eventually kill others to satiate their desire for blood

In 1992, Richard Noll, a psychologist and author of *Bizarre Diseases of the Mind,* described an unusual disorder in which a person craves blood, presumably to give him or her a special life force. He related it to the fact that some groups in history have believed that eating other living things and drinking blood give one special powers. Noll remembered a character in Bram Stoker's 1895 novel *Dracula.* R. M. Renfield ate flies, spiders, and birds because he thought he could capture some special life force. Noll thought that Renfield syndrome would be a proper name for this disorder.

WHAT IS RENFIELD SYNDROME?

Renfield syndrome, also known as clinical vampirism, is a rare condition in which the person drinks blood. The condition, which is usually found in males, is not recognized as a separate disorder in any edition of the *Diagnostic and Statistical Manual of Mental Disorders* (*DSM*) or in the International Classification of Diseases (ICD). It is usually thought to be associated with schizophrenia or paraphilia. Both of these are mental disorders: schizophrenia is a separation from reality, and paraphilia involves abnormal sex drives.

The idea of blood giving a special vital force has historical roots, along with the tales and literature of vampirism. Stories of vampires are especially known in Eastern Europe with a center in the mountains of Transylvania. Richard Vanden Bergh and John Kelly wrote one of the first psychiatric analyses of vampirism in the *Archives of General Psychiatry* in 1964. Most of the current cases involve criminal actions and are found in forensic literature.

The development of this extraordinary behavior appears to come in three stages:

Stage one: Some event in early childhood causes the child to get excited over the taste of blood. It might be that he cuts his finger and places it in his mouth to stop the bleeding. This behavior is called autohemophagia from the Greek words: *auto,* meaning "self;" *hemo,* meaning "blood;" and *phag,* meaning "to eat." The person may continue cutting himself and receiving some sort of satisfaction from the blood.

Stage two: This phase is called zoophagia, from the Greek words: *zo,* meaning "animal" and *phage* meaning "to eat." Not satisfied with her own blood, she begins to seek the blood of live animals. She may also get blood from a butcher or slaughterhouse.

Stage three: The person now graduates to humans. He may steal blood from a blood bank or hospital, or progress to getting blood from other humans. This stage is very dangerous, because he may kill to get the blood.

Several serial killers have performed vampire rituals on their victims. Serial killers Peter Kürten and Richard Trenton Chase were found to drink the blood of the people they murdered.

WHAT ARE THE SIGNS AND SYMPTOMS?

The main symptom of this disorder is the drinking of blood. Because it is not recognized as a separate condition, the diagnosis remains in limbo. However, lots of speculation about the cause does remain.

HOW IS IT DIAGNOSED?

The diagnosis of this rare condition is extremely difficult. A person with the condition may be traced to the committing of a crime, and consequently be in the legal system. The small amount of information and cases regarding Renfield syndrome is found in forensic literature.

WHAT IS THE TREATMENT?

No treatment exists for this condition, and there is a dearth of literature on the subject.

Dr. K. Gubb, in an article in the *South African Psychiatry Review* (2006) described the case history of Vlad B., a 36-year-old white male who came to their clinic for help. Since childhood, he had consumed animal blood. He was diagnosed with schizophrenia and felt completely out of control. His first exposure to vampirism was in the mental health system, when he met other men who were drinking blood. When he drank blood, he felt like he was empowered, and was in control of his out-of-control life. He had always been interested in mystery novels and crime shows. Treatment was very difficult, because when stripped of his vampirism, he lost control again; however, a therapist worked with him over a six-month period.

For Further Information

Jaffe, P. D., and F. DiCataldo. "Clinical Vampirism: Blending Myth and Reality." *Bulletin of the American Academy of Psychiatry and Law* 22 (4): 533–544, 1994.

Stockholm Syndrome: Bonding with Captors

- Hostages develop positive feelings about their captors and may even defend them afterwards
- First identified as a phenomenon in the 1970s, although it has likely existed for centuries

- FBI's database reveals that 8 percent of kidnapping victims and hostages show evidence of Stockholm syndrome
- May be similar to battered person syndrome or fraternity bonding by hazing

In 1972, a 19-year-old girl named Patty was kidnapped by a radical terrorist group called the Symbionese Liberation Army (SLU). She was seen on videotapes helping the SLA rob banks in San Francisco and other places, and even sent a tape recording under her new name Tania, telling of her support of the SLA cause. Patty's last name is Hearst, and she is the daughter of Randolph Hearst and an heir to the great newspaper empire run by the Hearst family. After her release from captivity, she described how she was bound, kept in a dark closet, and sexually abused. Afterwards at her trial, she told how, in order to survive, she had to comply and be helpful. Patty Hearst was a victim of Stockholm syndrome.

WHAT IS STOCKHOLM SYNDROME?

Stockholm syndrome is a psychological phenomenon in which a hostage or hostages develop empathy and feeling for their captors. Afterwards, they may even become concerned for their safety or defend them at their trial. In order to defend oneself, the person identifies with their captor or captors, interpreting any little kindness as reason to hold positive feelings toward that captor.

In August 1973, a man wielding a submachine gun burst into the Sveriges Kreditbanken in Stockholm, Sweden. Jan-Erik Olsson took four hostages and demanded the release of a friend who was in prison, $700,000, a getaway car, and the hostages as a shield. The authorities gave him all his demands, except using the hostages as a shield.

While in the bank vault with the robber, the hostages formed a strange bond with their captor. He did little favors for them; he gave his coat to one who was cold and let one who complained of claustrophobia while in the vault walk around the bank. These kindnesses were interpreted as gracious and good behavior, because they knew he had their lives in his hands. As the days wore on, the hostages began to fear for the safety of their captors and trusted them more than the police. After about 130 hours, the police threw tear gas into the vault and were able to subdue the criminals. Afterwards, the prisoners had only good things to say about their capturers. One of the women eventual married Olsson after his release from prison. In 1974, because of the unusual reactions of the prisoners, psychiatrist Frank Ochberg gave capture-bonding the name "Stockholm Syndrome."

Some historians trace the mindset of compliance back through history. Marauding bands would capture other tribes and carry off women, who became identified with the group. Many such stories are told of white women who were captured by Native Americans and adopted their way of life.

Some mental health workers compare this type of thinking to battered-person syndrome, in which women or men stay with a spouse who harasses, beats, threatens, or abuses them in some way. They develop strong emotional ties with those abusers and will defend their actions. This may explain why many battered spouses refuse to press charges against the abuser. This same type of thought has been seen in many other instances, such as concentration camps and prison camps, and during fraternity hazing and military basic training.

WHAT ARE THE SIGNS AND SYMPTOMS?

Persons who find themselves in this situation usually experience isolation and loneliness along with abuse. They may begin to think that they will never escape, and thus must comply with the demands of the captors. Psychiatrists have outlined the following four conditions that enable the captive to comply:

- **They believe the captors will and can kill them.** Olsson in Stockholm shot a male prisoner in the leg to show the police how much danger the captors were in. The man thanked him for not killing him, and that the leg wound was only superficial.
- **They are isolated from anyone but their captors.** In 1988, a 10-year-old girl from Austria was captured. She reappeared as an 18-year-old in 2006. She was kept in a basement room in the captor's home all during those years. She later told the authorities how fortunate she was because she was spared lots of the bad things that happen to young people—smoking, drinking, and hanging out with a bad crowd.
- They believe that escape is not possible. They even may begin to fear rescue attempts, because not only they could be injured, but their captor would also be hurt.
- They believe that any small act of kindness reflects genuine care of the captor.

HOW IS IT DIAGNOSED?

The diagnosis must come after some act of captivity endured by the person. The response of the person to this captivity would indicate whether or not the person has Stockholm syndrome.

WHAT IS THE TREATMENT?

The victims will be debriefed and offered psychological counseling. Many will realize how they developed the positive feelings as a coping mechanism. Patty Hearst later denounced the SLA, and said she had been brainwashed.

THE STRANGE CASE OF ELIZABETH SMART

On June 5, 2002 a 14-year-old girl, Elizabeth Smart was abducted from her bedroom in an upscale Salt Lake City home. Brian David Mitchell forced her at knifepoint to go with him. He and his wife took her to a makeshift campsite and there performed a fake marriage ceremony. She was then chained to a tree, starved, and repeatedly raped. She thought once that she heard a search party, but Mitchell threatened to kill her if she made any noise. She soon realized that crying and screaming would do no good, and that her only hope of survival was to comply with whatever they asked. Thus, in order to survive, she decided not to upset her captors, but to follow their commands. He then unchained her and took her to Salt Lake City in search of food and alcohol.

They moved around quite a bit. Once in California, she was approached by a police officer. She did not try to alert him as to who she was. She felt the threats to her and her family were so real that she could not chance it. Some people later criticized her for that—but the threats to her family became a strong bind to her captors. She realized that she would be a captive as long as they lived, and talked them into going back to Utah.

In the meantime, Smart's sister, who had also been in the bedroom, recognized the voice of the man as someone who had done work at their house. She was able to describe him to a police sketch artist. The picture was blasted on television. Several people spotted them in Sandy, Utah, and after nine months as a captive, Smart was reunited with her family.

Seven years later, she testified against Mitchell in court, where he received a life sentence. Since then, Smart has started a foundation to help prevent crimes against children and to help victims of sexual abuse. She has also married, and is trying to live a normal life.

For Further Information

Borst, Kelsi. *Stockholm Syndrome*. Bloomington, IN: AuthorHouse, 2008.

Trichotillomania: Pulling Hair

- Those afflicted compulsively pull out hair from the head or body
- Related to obsessive compulsive disorders
- May affect as much as 4 percent of the population
- Women are four times more likely to have the disorder than men

Several videos and television programs have focused on people who have an unusual disorder. They pull out their own hair, eyebrows, or body hair. Jennifer Raikes produced a documentary film called *Bad Hair Life* that explored trichotillomania. The film won numerous awards, including an International Health & Medical Media

Award for the best portrayal of a psychiatric condition. She tells about people who put bandages over their fingers, wear gloves on their hands, or don toboggan caps in both summer and winter. Some have tried all kinds of rewards and punishments, including punching themselves every time they pull their hair. Nothing seems to work. Jennifer herself struggles with trichotillomania, a condition in which she has an uncontrollable urge to pull out her own hair.

WHAT IS TRICHOTILLOMANIA?

Trichotillomania is a condition in which the person pulls out hair, eyelashes, eyebrows, or hair in other body parts, causing obvious bald patches. It is classified as similar to obsessive compulsive disorder (OCD), because the person does not have control over the urge to pull out hair. Other similar disorders include nail biting, skin picking, tic disorders, and eating disorders. Without treatment, it can become a chronic condition that will come and go throughout life.

The word "trichotillomania" comes from three Greek words: *tricho* meaning "hair," *tillo* meaning "pull," and *mania* meaning "a madness for" or "a desire for." Some individuals describe that they feel an unusual tension before pulling the hair out, and that that feeling is released or satisfied once the act is done. Some say they do not realize that they are pulling or twisting their hair. Often, it is not a focused or conscious act, but occurs in a mindless, thoughtless trance.

Hair pulling has a long history in scientific literature. In 1885 the French dermatologist Francois Henri Hallopeau (1842–1919) coined the term trichotillomania. The condition was first listed as a mental disorder in the *Diagnostic and Statistical Manual of Mental Disorders* (*DSM*) in 1987. It is also listed in the European International Classification of Diseases (ICD), in Chapter 5, "Mental and Behavioral Disorders." Because this condition may be more common than affecting only 4 percent of the population, and the habit itself is so destructive to the appearance and self-esteem, it is included as one of the unusual mental disorders.

Although the exact cause may not be known, one theory, called the neurocognitive model, believes that it may be related to abnormalities in brain pathways that regulate emotion, habit formation, movement, and impulse control. Some people may have depression, anxiety, or other stress disorders. Multiple genes may also be involved.

WHAT ARE THE SIGNS AND SYMPTOMS?

Trichotillomania may be present in infants and young children; however, the peak age of onset is nine to 13. For adults, the symptoms usually begin before the age of 17. The person will have patches of hair that are missing from the scalp, which gives an uneven or bald appearance. The individual may constantly tug or pull at the hair. This person may also pick at other hairy areas, such as eyebrows, eyelashes, or body hair. He or she may have a sense of relief from stress and a sense of satisfaction after the hair pulling. Associated with hair pulling are feelings of depression, anxiety, and poor self-image. If the person eats or chews on the hair, he or she may suffer some type of bowel blockage.

Two subtypes are identified: automatic and focused. Children are most often in the automatic group. They will unconsciously pull out their hair and not remember doing so. The second group of individuals are focused or conscious, and have certain events or rituals for pulling hair. They may have usual times for hair pulling. It could be when the person is in a quiet, sedentary environment. A common time is when lying in bed trying to fall asleep. Other times include reading, working at the computer, watching TV, talking on the telephone, riding in a car, using the bathroom, or listening in class. To help in the diagnosis and treatment, knowing the subtype is important.

HOW IS IT DIAGNOSED?

The actual diagnosis may be difficult because the person is ashamed and does not want to admit there is a problem. The diagnosis is based on the symptoms. If the person has patches of baldness that cannot be explained by other diseases, there is a likelihood of the disorder. There is no specific test.

WHAT IS THE TREATMENT?

Age is a factor in treatment. Young children will probably outgrow the problem with simple encouragement. When working with young adults, it is essential to help them be aware of the problem. The following treatments may be used:

- **Behavior modification programs.** One major type is called habit reversal training, which means the person replaces a bad habit with one that is not harmful.
- **Biofeedback therapies.** These include cognitive-behavioral methods and hypnosis.
- **Medication.** Some people have been treated with clomipramine, a tricyclic antidepressant. Medications are not the first line of treatment, and have mixed results with individuals.
- **Support groups and sharing.** Both meeting and online groups have great benefit for people with the disorder. A support group called the Trichotillomania Learning Center (TLC) provides education, information, and encouragement.

For Further Information

Chamberlain, S. R., L. Menzies, B. J. Sahakian, and N. A. Fineberg. "Lifting the Veil on Trichotillomania." *American Journal of Psychiatry* 164 (4): 568–74, 2007.

Hennerberg, Gary. *Urges: Hope and Inspiration for People with Trichotillomania.* Amazon. com (CreateSpace): Doses of Comfort Publishing, 2009.

PART III

UNUSUAL ENVIRONMENTAL DISEASES AND DISORDERS

WHAT YOU SHOULD KNOW ABOUT ENVIRONMENTAL DISEASES AND DISORDERS

Environmental disorders are those that are attributed to surroundings or environment. Some of the disorders, such as stachybotrys and vibrio, are actually infectious diseases, but they are included in this section because of their strong connection to a particular environment. A genetic component may be involved for those who are predisposed to certain conditions. For example, for those who are predisposed to certain kinds of cancer, cigarette smoking, an environmental factor, may be involved. A large number of factors may be involved in causes of nonhereditary disease. These could include stress diet, exposure to toxins, certain pathogens, radiation, and the chemicals in all kinds of products, from household cleaners to cosmetics.

The disorders included in this section are not the ordinary ones. Although some of them may be common, they are not well known, or are misunderstood. Some of them have a mythology that surrounds them.

Some of the disorders are strictly related to environment or environmental conditions. These include altitude sickness and frostbite. Several conditions relate to ingesting metals or chemicals. These include silver (argyria, which causes blue skin), pneumoconiosis, and thalidomide. Some of the disorders are the results of encounters with animals such as bats or jellyfish, or insects such as the brown recluse spider or *Solenopsis invicta*, the fire ant.

Two digital age conditions are included, computer vision syndrome and tech neck. Although these may not be uncommon, the symptoms are not recognized as a disorder, and how to treat or avoid these conditions are not generally known or understood.

For Further Information

Barceloux, Donald G. *Medical Toxicology of Natural Substances: Foods, Fungi, Medicinal Herbs, Plants, and Venomous Animals.* New York: John Wiley and Sons, 2008.

Nagami, Pamela. *Bitten: True Medical Stories of Bites and Stings.* New York: St. Martin's Griffin, 2005.

Norman, Robert. *The Blue Man and Other Stories of the Skin.* Berkeley, CA: University of California Press, 2014.

Paul, Annie Murphy. *Origins: How the Nine Months Before Birth Shape the Rest of Our Lives.* New York: Free Press, 2011.

Altitude Sickness: Those Beautiful High Mountains Can Make You Ill

- Prevalence: Mild altitude sickness; fairly common, and may affect over 20 percent of people who go above 8,000 feet
- High altitude stresses the body through dehydration
- Can be potentially life-threatening in its more severe forms
- Treatment usually involves supplemental oxygen, and descending below 8,000 feet

When you think of mountain climbing, you think of the rush and thrill of reaching the top and looking victoriously down upon the world. But did you realize that these adventurers may be subject to a debilitating and possibly lethal condition—altitude sickness?

This mysterious illness strikes suddenly, and experts disagree on whom it may hit, and when. The illness begins with "flu-like symptoms" or other nonspecific symptoms. It can also lead to the fatal conditions called high altitude pulmonary edema (HAPE) or high cerebral edema (HACE).

WHAT IS ALTITUDE SICKNESS?

Altitude sickness occurs for some people when they travel above 8,000 feet. Symptoms vary, but generally include severe headache and malaise. Most cases are mild, but under certain circumstances, cases can be fatal.

Mountain climbing and hiking, as well as traveling to places of high elevation, are popular activities. The high-altitude environment places numerous stresses on the human body. These include cold temperatures, low humidity that can lead to dehydration, increased exposure to ultraviolet rays, and decreased air pressure, with less oxygen in the air. The thin mountain air can lead to a condition called "hypoxia," which is the primary concern. The word "hypoxia" comes from two Greek root words: *hypo*, meaning "under" and *oxy*, meaning "oxygen."

According to the Centers for Disease Control and Prevention (CDC), the height that appears to be the dividing line is 8,000 feet or 2,500 meters. Camping and hiking in such areas as the Rocky Mountains in Colorado, or visits to high-altitude countries such as Bolivia, Ecuador, Peru, Tibet, or Nepal, are likely settings for altitude sickness. Most people live and work at much lower altitudes, and when one travels above that critical line, the body must adjust. The human body generally can tolerate moderate hypoxia if the person ascends the mountain slowly over a three to five day period, and does not over exert. Mild altitude sickness is fairly common, and may affect over 20 percent of people.

WHAT ARE THE SIGNS AND SYMPTOMS?

The signs and symptoms are nonspecific, and vary with the individual. Some people may just get a simple headache when driving through a mountain pass. Headaches are probably the chief complaint, and for more than about half of the individuals, the headache goes away when the person become acclimated to the new atmospheric conditions.

There are three types of altitude sickness: acute mountain sickness (AMS), high-altitude cerebral edema (HACE), and high-altitude pulmonary edema (HAPE).

Acute mountain sickness is the least dangerous, affecting over half of people who mountain climb. Most people describe it as a throbbing headache that gets worse at night, then continues the next morning. Some have described it as being like a "severe hangover." Likewise, other conditions may vary. The person may not want to eat and may be sick to his stomach and want to vomit. The individual becomes very weak and is dizzy or lightheaded. She may have insomnia, or want to sleep all the time. Some people experience shortness of breath, nosebleed, the feeling of pins and needles pricking the skin, rapid pulse, or excessive flatulence. Usually the condition resolves after 24 to 72 hours of acclimatizing, or descending to a lower altitude. And mysteriously, sometimes the symptoms do not occur until the person has descended to a lower altitude.

High-altitude cerebral edema (HACE) occurs when edema or swelling begins in the cerebral area of the brain. The symptoms include headache that does not respond to painkillers, an unsteady gait, and severe nausea. The person may lose consciousness or in an extreme case, may hemorrhage in the retina of the eye. The person should descend to a lower altitude immediately. Although physicians do not always know the cause, they suspect that the blood vessels in the brain dilate in response to the lower oxygen, which causes greater blood flow and increased pressure in the arteries. Coma or death may result.

High-altitude Pulmonary Edema (HAPE) has more specific symptoms. Because of the lung implications, those with HAPE may have a dry cough, which is similar to bronchitis, fever, shortness of breath even when resting, and frothy pink sputum. The cause appears to be the opposite of the cause of HACE. In this type, blood vessels in the lung constrict, which in turn puts extra pressure on the heart to pump. HAPE is possibly more fatal than HACE.

HOW IS IT DIAGNOSED?

If the person has been in any of the areas of high altitude and comes down with an illness, the doctor can suspect the problem may be related to altitude. Oxygen is essential to sustain mental and physical energy. As altitude increases, available oxygen drops. How fast the person climbs, and the physical activity, along with dehydration due to loss of water vapor from the lungs, may contribute to the symptoms of altitude sickness. Experts disagree on whom it will strike and when. No specific type of person appears more susceptible. Body fitness does not appear to be a factor, although some sources say genetics, advanced age, previous medical conditions, and obesity may be involved. Children as well as adults, and men as well as women, may be affected.

WHAT IS THE TREATMENT?

Knowing the potential consequences of altitude sickness is important for mountain climbers and for travelers to high countries. If the person only has a headache, he or she should take a mild pain reliever; however, if other symptoms such as nausea or confusion are present, he can suspect acute altitude sickness. Those traveling at these heights should know that it is essential to watch one's companions for any sign of disorientation. Anyone who is hiking or camping who develops such symptoms should be slowly moved back down to lower elevations. Those who are in a city that has high elevations and who observe persistent symptoms should contact a health care professional.

Here are some tips for those who are mountain climbing or camping at high elevations:

- Before you begin, know the elevation of the place you are ascending to.
- Ascend the mountain gradually, climbing in a progressive manner; it is suggested that you plan an extra day for acclimatization for every 3,300 feet.
- Do only mild exercise for the first 48 hours that you are hiking or climbing.
- Drink plenty of fluids and do not drink alcohol, or take sleeping pills or pain medications.
- Consider asking your doctor about the prescription drug acetazolamide (Diamox®)

TIPS FOR TRAVELING TO HIGH ELEVATION LOCATIONS:

- Before you go, visit a doctor or nurse who specializes in travel information. These practitioners can be found at county health departments, or you can go online to the Centers for Disease Control and Prevention website for information.
- Know the elevation of your destination.
- Understand the importance of keeping hydrated. Remember, the thin air causes body moisture to evaporate, leaving one dehydrated.
- Wear hats and use sun protection. Even if the temperature is cold or if it is cloudy, the sun's radiation is powerful at high elevations.
- If you know you have a problem with altitude sickness, consider asking your doctor about the prescription drug acetazolamide (Diamox®).

For Further Information

Dremousis, Litsa. *Altitude Sickness.* Portland, OR: Instant Future Press, 2013.

PubMed Health. A service of the National Library of Medicine, National Institutes of Health. A.D.A.M. Medical Encyclopedia. https://www.nlm.nih.gov/medlineplus/encyclopedia .html.

Argyria: When a Person Turns Blue

- Accumulation of silver in the body causes skin to turn blue
- Two types: localized and universal
- Internal organs may also be affected
- Skin discoloration is very difficult to reverse

When Rosemary was 11, her mother told her doctor in Long Island that she always appeared to have a cold. The doctor prescribed nose drops containing silver. When she was in high school, a nun asked her, "Why are you that color?" She went to a dermatologist who diagnosed her with argyria, a permanent discoloration. She found the doctor in Long Island had read only the ads about the nose drops, and not the medical literature. Before the days of antibiotics, silver was popular for treatment, and is still used in certain alternative therapies.

WHAT IS ARGYRIA?

Argyria is a condition that results from prolonged exposure to silver, and makes the skin turn a bluish gray. The term "argyria" comes from the Greek word *argyros,* meaning "silver." The Romans adapted the word for silver as *argentium.* The chemical symbol for silver in the Periodic table is Ag, from argentium. The country Argentina was dubbed "the land of silver" because its name is derived from the word "argentium."

There are several ways that silver can get into the skin. Small particles may impregnate the skin of workers in certain occupations that deal with silver. Following are risk factors:

- Working in a silver mine
- Making silverware or using silver in electroplating of glass or china
- Photographic processing
- Certain surgical or dental procedures that use silver sutures
- Silver amalgam tattooing

- Acupuncture needles
- Silver earrings

The other risk factors involve people who take colloidal silver to treat an assortment of conditions.

WHAT ARE THE SIGNS AND SYMPTOMS?

The blue-grey patches may appear in localized areas on the skin, or it may be generalized. Following are the two types of argyria:

- **Localized.** This type is caused by topical treatments, such as nasal sprays containing silver compounds that affect the sensitive mucous membranes of the nose. Items such as tattoo colors that have a silver base and silver earrings may trigger a localized reaction.
- **Universal.** This type develops from long-term use of drugs that contain silver salts. Some of these are marketed on the internet for a variety of conditions, including cancer, AIDS, diabetes, arthritis, stomach and intestinal problems, and other conditions.

The universal type may not only affect the skin; the internal organs may also be laden with the deposits of silver.

HOW IS IT DIAGNOSED?

The color of the skin in patches or overall is a tell-tale clue. A physician will look at these patches under fluorescent X-ray. A biopsy of the area will indicate that excess silver has been deposited. A normal human being has about 1 milligram of silver in his or her body. However, the accumulation of 4 grams or more puts a person at risk for argyria.

WHAT IS THE TREATMENT?

The person must stop the exposure to silver, because continued use can lead to serious complications. However, once the skin patches or color has appeared, it is very difficult to reverse. Some doctors have had success treating localized patches with hydroquinone ointment or laser surgery. Patients with argyria are advised to limit their time in the sun and to always use sunscreen.

The history of medicine is dotted with silver as a treatment. Before antibiotics, it was used to treat a variety of infectious diseases. Since 1990, "colloidal silver" has been marketed as an alternative product. In 1999 the U.S. Food and Drug

---

FAMOUS ARGYRIA CASES

The Famous "Blue Man" from Ringling Brothers and Barnum & Bailey Circus. In the late nineteenth and the turn of the twentieth century, the Blue Man appeared in the circus "freak show" of Ringling Brothers and Barnum & Bailey Circus, known as "The Greatest Show on Earth." When he died in 1924, the body was sent to the morgue of the medical examiner in New York. His skin was a deep blue, almost black, and so were his lips and tongue. The white of his eyes were blue. He had ingested silver nitrate to keep the color of his skin so he could be in the show. The autopsy showed that even his brain was blue. However, the pathologist also determined that he did not die from argyria, but from pneumonia.

Candidate for Montana Senate. Libertarian Stan Jones ran for a U.S. Senate seat for Montana in 2002 and 2006. He had started using homemade silver in 2000 during the "Y2K scare," thinking that antibiotics would soon not be available. His blue skin got a lot of media attention, but he lost the race in both years.

Paul Karason of Oregon. In 1998, Karason saw an ad in a New Age magazine promising health and rejuvenation through colloidal silver. He made his own suspension, and drank 10 ounces a day. His arthritis was gone, but his skin turned blue. He hoped it would fade, but it never did. He later died of a heart attack, not related to argyria.

Administration (FDA) issued a warning that all over-the-counter (OTC) drug products containing colloidal silver ingredients for internal and external use are not recognized as safe and effective, and are misbranded.

Colloidal silver is processed so that silver of a specific particle size is in suspension. Some sites on the internet market home kits that show people how to make their own colloidal suspensions using silver and distilled water. These are especially dangerous, because the size of the particles may affect the skin.

For Further Information

Hill, John. *Colloidal Silver Medical Uses, Toxicology & Manufacture.* Ranier, WA: Clear Springs Press, 2009.

Brown Recluse Bite: The Spider with the Violin on Its Back

- Violin pattern found on the backs of most brown recluses
- Likes secluded spots; may be inside houses

- Bites can cause serious skin damage
- Severe cases may require intensive treatment, including hyperbaric oxygen and surgical excision

Ben, a 65-year-old Florida resident, was cleaning out a closet that that had been accumulating things for years. He picked up a stack of clothes and felt something like a bite on the underside of his upper right arm. The bite was not really painful, but he did capture a brown spider with something that looked like a violin on its back. About 24 hours later, the area began to hurt, and he went to the emergency room. They put some ice on the area, gave him a tetanus shot, prescribed something for pain, and sent him home. Three days later the wound had turned into a saucer-sized open ulcer, which showed a red, white, and blue area. So he returned again and was hospitalized. He stayed for three days to combat his reaction to the bite of the brown recluse spider.

Although this spider's habitat is in one specific region, they may occasionally show up in other regions.

WHAT IS THE BROWN RECLUSE SPIDER?

The scientific name is *Loxosceles reclusa,* but it is commonly called the brown recluse or violin spider. These spiders, which are only a little larger than a U.S. penny, pack a venomous bite. They range in color from a brown cream to a dark brown, but have black markings on their back that look like a fiddle or violin. Like other spiders, the recluse has two body parts, the cephalothorax, which is the head and chest fused on one body part, and the abdomen. Eight legs are on the cephalothorax. But a major difference exists between this and other spiders. Most spiders have eight eyes; the brown recluse has only six.

The recluse builds asymmetrical or orbed webs that are located in woodpiles, rotting bark, sheds, attics, basements, shoes, dressers, toilets, cardboard boxes, behind pictures, closets, garages, cellars, unused beds, and other places. You will not see them on a web or spinning to catch insects. They adapt well to the indoors and find isolated places in houses, where there is not much activity. It is not an aggressive spider and usually bites only when intruded upon. For example, the body of a person in bed rolls over on the spider, or it is tangled in a towel, in work gloves, or in a sleeper. Its habitat is about 15 states in the South, Midwest, and Southwest.

True to its name, "recluse," the spider is rarely seen during daylight hours. The egg sacs produce several eggs over a period of two to three months with about 50 eggs in each sac. The little spiders take about a year to mature.

Why the bite of this small spider can inflict such damage is not completely understood. The venom has an enzyme sphingomyelinase D, which attacks and dissolves the membranes of the cells. This enzyme, along with several others, sets off a chain of chemical reactions that turns the person's immune system against itself. The white blood cells that normally act to destroy invaders implode, and release other invaders that destroy the patient's own flesh. Clots then form inside the vessels that nourish the skin, and a deep ulcer forms. The reaction takes several weeks.

The bites are painful and debilitating, but usually are not life-threatening, unless located in a place such as the neck of an adult, or anywhere on a very young child, an older person, or a person with an already compromised immune system.

WHAT ARE THE SIGNS AND SYMPTOMS?

The bite may not be felt, but a typical scenario may be similar to the one that Ben experienced. After about a day, the person may develop an ulcer that shows a distinct red, white, and blue pattern. This is called necrotic arachnidism. Arachnid is the scientific name for the spider, and necrosis is the deterioration of tissue. When looking from the outer edge to the center, there is first a red circle of inflammation, then inside that is a smaller ring of white tissue in which the blood flow to the skin is blocked, and in the center is a blue circle of dying tissue. The person may now have fever, severe pain, and a red rash over his or her body. With treatment, the ulcer may heal, but will leave a scar.

HOW IS IT DIAGNOSED?

The diagnosis may be missed at first because at the beginning, it appears like other bite marks, or may not even be felt. The telling signs for diagnosis include the red, white, and blue circles, the pain, and the rash that develops over the body.

WHAT IS THE TREATMENT?

First aid involves washing the area with soap and water, then using an ice pack to control inflammation. The recommended time for ice application is 10 minutes on and 10 minutes, off until medical treatment is available. It helps if the spider is caught and identified. The area will be immobilized and a tetanus shot given. Various therapies have been used with varying degrees of success, including hyperbaric oxygen, dapsone, antihistamines, antibiotics, surgical excision, and antivenom. However, most cases are self-healing, and the person is usually given instructions for outpatient palliative care.

For Further Information

Nagami, Pamela. Bitten: *True Medical Stories of Bites and Stings.* New York: St. Martin's Griffin, 2004.

Computer Vision Syndrome (CVS): Eyes and the Digital Age

- Also called digital eye strain
- Affects about 90 percent of people who spend three hours or more a day at a computer or other digital devices
- Digital devices exhibit a number of features that make the eyes work harder
- Has surpassed carpal tunnel syndrome and tendinitis as the most common repetitive strain injury among workers

Nancy, a college student and single mother, was so proud of her new smart phone. It was the only digital device that she owned, and she spent many hours on it. She even wrote term papers on the handy little instrument. However, one morning she woke up and could not read the numbers on the digital clock. The doctor said that the constant straining of her eyes had caused an inflammation of the nerves called neuritis. She had to take six weeks away from the phone and make plans to get a computer that had a large screen and higher resolution. For the first time, Nancy heard about a condition common to those who work on digital devices, called computer vision syndrome.

Computer vision syndrome is relatively new condition that few people are aware of. Technology is important in the lives of people today, and its use is more and more sophisticated. This condition is one that is unique because of its relationship to digital use and the digital age.

WHAT IS COMPUTER VISION SYNDROME?

Computer vision syndrome (CVS) is a temporary condition that describes a group of eye-related problems that affect people who use certain electronic digital devices for long periods of time. Although the computer and smart phones are the most common sources of the problem, other digital devices such as digital game systems, tablet or eReaders, and television may also affect the eyes and other body areas.

Anyone who uses these devices for a long period of time is at risk for digital eye strain. It has little to do with age or experience in using the devices, but is related to the amount of time one spends on the computer. Kids who play computer games for hours or who use computers throughout the day in their classes may also have CVS.

Working with any of these digital devices requires that the eyes are in continual movement. This movement is controlled by muscles that are put in constant motion. The computer screen itself presents a challenge. It adds contrast, glare, and flicker. The characters on the computer are made up of little dots or squares called pixels. These dots display letters that are not sharply defined and not uniformly dense. This problem of display is not present when reading print on a page.

In addition, certain other physical things may come into play. These include poor lighting, excessive glare on the screen, sitting at an unusual distance, or having poor posture. Viewing distances and angles for computer work may put additional strain on the muscles. The person may be working in bed or working with the laptop on the lap while viewing television. Just because a person has prescription eyeglasses that are used for reading does not mean that the glasses are suitable for reading on a computer screen. Some individuals hold their heads at unusual angles or bend towards the screen to see clearly. These environmental constraints can add to visual demands.

WHAT ARE THE SIGNS AND SYMPTOMS?

CVS is not just one specific eye problem, but covers a host of troublesome symptoms. The most common eye problems include eyestrain, in which the eyes become red and irritated, headaches, blurred vision, double vision, vertigo or dizziness, and dry eye, a chronic condition in which the eye does not produce the proper amount of moisture. In addition to the eye, part of the syndrome can include shoulder and neck pain and fatigue.

Other conditions may aggravate and evoke CVS. If an individual has other eye problems such as farsightedness and astigmatism, which are not corrected, the condition may escalate. Changes within the eyes due to age, a condition known as presbyopia, may affect those over 40.

HOW IS IT DIAGNOSED?

According to the Vision Council, a nonprofit organization in the optical industry, digital eye strain is now the most common computer-related injury, supplanting carpal tunnel syndrome and tendinitis. When a person goes for an eye exam, he or she needs to inform the doctor of the amount of computer use. The doctor will take a patient history, noting general health, medications taken that may affect eye performance, and other environmental factors. The doctor will then make visual acuity measurements and test for eye problems, such as nearsightedness, farsightedness, or astigmatism. He or she will then test to see how well the eyes focus, move, and work together.

WHAT IS THE TREATMENT?

The doctor will probably give the person some tips for working with digital devices (see sidebar). If one already has prescription lenses, the doctor may find that the regular glasses are not adequate for computer work. Prescribing lenses with a special design, power, or tint may help the person avoid eye strain. For those who have more severe problems, vision therapy may be prescribed to help train the eye and brain to work effectively together.

TIPS FOR WORKING WITH THE COMPUTER

- **1.20-20-20.** Many eye care providers promote the 20-20-20 rule. That means for every 20 minutes that a person is on the computer, he or she should look away for 20 seconds at some object that is about 20 feet away. This simple exercise relaxes eye muscles and keeps them focused when viewing close objects.
- **Blink.** Blinking stimulates tear production and avoids developing dry eye. Blinking helps keep the front surface of the eye moist.
- **Rest breaks.** About every 20 to 30 minutes, get up and take a brief break from the screen.
- **Change the screen.** Increasing the size of the font may help a person keep from squinting. Also, make changes in the brightness and contrast settings. High resolution screens may be bought.
- **Look down.** Recommended location of the screen should be about 4 or 5 inches below eye level from the center of the screen. The screen should be about 20 to 28 inches from the eyes.
- **Reading materials.** Many people must use materials for reference as they work on the screen. If these are lying flat or in an awkward place, a person must constantly move the head to look at the document. The material should be located above the keyboard and above the monitor. A document holder may position the material so that movements of the head are reduced.
- **Light.** Make sure there is no glare from overhead lights or windows. Blinds or drapes on the window can reduce light. Use a low wattage bulb near the computer. To cut glare, invest in an anti-glare screen.
- **Sit up.** The office chair is one of the most important pieces of furniture in an office. It should be comfortably padded and conform to the body. Adjust the height of the seat so that the feet can fit comfortably on the floor.

For Further Information

Yan, Zheng, Liang Hu, Hao Chen, and Fan Lu. 2008. "Computer Vision Syndrome: A Widely Spreading but Largely Unknown Epidemic among Computer Users." *Computers in Human Behavior* 24 (5): 2026–2042.

DES Sons and Daughters: When a Mother's Pregnancy Affects Successive Generations

- DES was used to prevent miscarriage
- Prevalence: Between 1940 and 1971, between 5 to 10 million Americans were exposed to DES

- DES daughters over 40 are twice as likely to have breast cancer
- DES sons are at greater risk for testicular cancer

Ellie, 69, has had a very aggressive form of breast cancer, several miscarriages, and many reproductive problems. She is not the only member of her family with medical issues. Her sister died at 41 with uterine cancer, and now her 41-year-old daughter has vaginal adenocarcinoma. Her mother, who was a nurse, told her that in the 1940s, she was given a hopeful new drug called diethylstilbestrol or DES, to prevent miscarriage.

When Ellie was told by her doctor about the generational effects of DES, she reacted with shock and disbelief. How could a medication that her mother took now be affecting herself, her daughter, and even future generations? Now she is an advocate for DES daughters and sons, encouraging them to know the facts and to seek the best care from doctor specializing in DES issues. Because of the continuing questions about the sons and daughters of those who took DES during pregnancy, it is included as one of the unusual environmental disorders.

WHAT IS DES SONS AND DAUGHTERS?

DES sons and daughters are the offspring of women who took diethylstilbestrol (DES), a synthetic form of estrogen, which was first made in 1938. From about 1940 to 1970, it was given to pregnant women to prevent miscarriage, premature labor, and other complications of pregnancy. In 1971, DES began to be connected to some cancer problems in women. Other health problems were then found in daughters and sons of women who took DES during pregnancies; studies of the grandchildren of these women are just beginning.

In 1938 Leon Goldberg, a graduate student at Oxford University, synthesized a form of nonsteroidal estrogen that was found to be an endocrine disruptor, a chemical that acts upon the hormones of the body. As a disruptor, it was supposed to be a miracle drug given to women between 1940 and 1971 to prevent premature labor, miscarriage, and other complications of pregnancy. It was also considered to be a growth hormone, and was used as a supplement in cattle feed and for treatment for certain types of breast and prostate cancers. In the 1950s, studies showed that it did not help the complications of pregnancy. However, in 1971, researchers found a certain type of cancer in the cervix and vagina called adenocarcinoma. The U.S. Food and Drug Administration told physicians in 1971 not to prescribe DES to pregnant women. However, it was continued in Europe until 1978. DES continued to be used for many treatments until the last manufacturer stopped making it in 1997.

WHAT ARE THE SIGNS AND SYMPTOMS?

Of the 3 million women who were prescribed DES during pregnancy between 1940 and 1970, many were shown to have had a modest risk of breast cancer and death. However, serious problems appear to rise in the first generation of both sons and daughters of those whose mothers took DES during pregnancy.

DES Daughters

In 1971 A. L. Herbst et al. published a study in the *New England Journal of Medicine* describing the appearance of adenocarcinoma of the vagina in seven of eight young women whose mothers had taken DES. The DES daughters were found to have about 40 times the risk of developing clear cell adenocarcinoma of the lower genital tract than those who were unexposed; about 1 in 1000 DES daughters developed these cancers. In addition, the daughters also were at risk for cervical cancer, and at an increased risk for an aggressive form of breast cancer.

Hoover et al., in a 2011 *New England Journal of Medicine* article, described how about 2 percent of a large cohort of DES daughters developed this very aggressive form of breast cancer, and that the risk increases in women over 40. The same study found infertility, spontaneous abortion, preterm delivery, ectopic pregnancy, preeclampsia, stillbirth, early menopause, and loss of second-trimester pregnancy were adverse effects of daughters of women exposed to DES. There may also be an increased risk of uterine fibroids.

DES Sons

DES-exposed males had an increased risk of testicular cancer and other types of growths and cysts. The American Association of Clinical Endocrinologists has documented a connection between prenatal exposure to DES and low testosterone levels. In addition, researcher Dr. Scott Kerlin documented for 15 years a high prevalence of individuals with male-to-female transsexual, transgender, and intersected problems. However, other studies have not confirmed this finding.

Second Generation

Now researchers are looking at the second generation. These are children of men and women who were exposed in utero, and the grandchildren of those given the original doses. These studies are important, because it may show that the way genes behave, and not only how the genes themselves are affected. These changes are called epigenetic changes. Some studies of animal models do support the idea that changes are actually made in the DNA, and are potentially heritable to subsequent generations.

HOW IS IT DIAGNOSED?

Diagnosis of this condition may be difficult if there is no knowledge of family history. The affected person may not be aware that that his or her mother took DES when pregnant. If there is a family history, both sons and daughters need to be aware that they are at risk for aggressive cancers, and let their health provider know.

WHAT IS THE TREATMENT?

DES sons and daughters should be aware of the risks. However, people in the 1940s did not know there was a problem, and many of the daughters were not aware their mothers had taken DES. The DES was given under many different names and in several forms. There were pills, creams, and vaginal suppositories. Researchers are continuing to study the sons and daughters as they move into their later years. Treatment varies according to the effect of the cancer, but usually surgery is necessary to remove cancerous growths.

For Further Information

DES Action USA. http://www.desaction.org/.

Langston, Nancy. *Toxic Bodies: Hormone Disruptors and the Legacy of DES*. New Haven, CT: Yale University Press, 2010.

Frostbite: A Cold Weather Problem

- A type of cold injury that causes localized damage
- Cells of skin and tissues freeze
- Four degrees of severity, each with varying degrees of pain
- Severe frostbite may require amputation

On January 28, 2014, a massive snow storm struck Atlanta, Georgia, a city that usually does not get such severe weather. Although there had been some warning, schools in the area were open, and it was not until noon that children were sent home on school buses. What school officials did not know, was that everyone else was leaving offices, causing a major traffic jam on Atlanta roads. People were stuck for hours in their cars and buses, in the cold. Fortunately, the people who were stalled in traffic for hours had only minor cold trauma, a condition called frostnip.

WHAT IS FROSTBITE?

Frostbite occurs when a person is exposed to very cold temperatures and certain underlying body tissues freeze. The fluid part is the medium for circulating several types of blood cells and many other life-sustaining cells; at or below 0°C (32°F), the blood vessels start to constrict. This constriction is a protective device, so that the temperature in the body core can be preserved. Clots occur in the blood vessels that then keep oxygen from reaching the tissues. The lack of oxygen causes death to the affected area. Although any body part may be affected, the most common areas are the fingers, feet, toes, nose, and ears.

The prolonged exposure to cold temperatures causes circulation to be directed to the body core. Not only is the cold temperature a factor, a strong wind may also add to the effect of the cold. Usually it occurs when there is long exposure; however, it can occur following brief exposure to very cold temperatures. In addition, some people may be more likely to develop symptoms.

A long list of factors may add to the risk: medicines called beta-blockers, circulation problems such as peripheral artery disease or Raynaud's phenomenon, tight clothing or boots, fatigue, alcohol use, or diabetes. Smoking constricts circulation to the extremities, putting smokers at greater risk. Children and older adults appear to react more readily to the cold; however, most cases of frostbite occur between the ages of 30 and 49.

There are some other happenings not related to weather that can cause frostbite. Examples are treatment with liquid nitrogen for certain skin cancers, parasitic conditions, or prolonged contact with aerosols.

WHAT ARE THE SIGNS AND SYMPTOMS?

In addition to frostbite, a person who has been exposed to cold may also have lowered body temperature or hypothermia, a very serious medical condition. It is wise to check for those symptoms and treat those people first. A person who is experiencing cold injury may not be aware that anything is wrong, because the body part is numb.

Following are the four degrees of cold injury relating to frostbite:

- **First degree or frostnip.** The area begins to itch and feel like pins and needles are pricking the skin; the area begins to throb and hurt. Color changes progress from white to red with yellow patches as the area becomes quite numb.
  The person may not feel the touch of another person. If the person receives treatment, only the top layers of skin are affected, so the skin will probably not be permanently damaged; however, the person may have a long-term sensitivity to cold and even heat.

- **Second degree or superficial frostbite.** If the exposure to cold is continued, the skin of the affected area may become hard and dark. In a few days, blisters may develop. Although most of these situations may heal within a month or so, the area may still be sensitive to both heat and cold.
- **Third degree or deep frostbite.** The person has been exposed for a prolonged period of time. The entire area of muscles, tendons, blood vessels, and nerves are frozen. The skin feels waxy and hard. The affected areas develop purplish blisters that are black and filled with blood. Because the nerves are damaged, there is no feeling in the area.
- **Fourth degree or extreme frostbite.** The area becomes infected with gangrene, a potentially life-threatening condition that occurs when body tissues die. Gangrene develops when the circulation is cut off for a long period of time. If the area does not receive treatment, the toes or fingers may fall off. This degree of damage is difficult to assess, and it may take months before surgeons can remove the dead tissue.

HOW IS IT DIAGNOSED?

If the person was exposed to the cold, he or she will be evaluated on the degree of injury. The cases will be placed in one of the four categories.

WHAT IS THE TREATMENT?

The person must have access to a warm, stable environment. If the skin area is warmed and then refrozen, serious damage may occur. Warming should be gradual. Put the affected area in warm water until the color returns. Never use hot water, and do not put the person near direct heat, such as a fire. Remember, he or she has no feeling and can be injured.

Other suggestions for treatment include the following:

- Do not rub or massage the area. One old "remedy" was to rub the area with snow; this can be extremely damaging.
- Do not break the blisters on the skin.
- Do not let the person walk on or use the affected area.
- Do not allow the person to smoke or drink alcoholic beverages, because these activities are depressants that decrease circulation.
- Get emergency help if numbness or sustained pain remains after warming

One of the best strategies for treating frostbite is to avoid it, if possible. Be aware that wet clothes, high winds, and poor circulation can make you a casualty. In cold climates, wear mittens, not gloves, waterproof and water-resistant layered clothing, two pairs of socks, and a hat or scarf that covers the ears, to avoid heat loss through the scalp.

For Further Information

Roche-Nagle, G., D. Murphy, A. Collins, and S. Sheehan. 2008. "Frostbite: Management Options." *European Journal of Emergency Medicine* 15 (3): 173–5.

Histoplasmosis: Cave Disease

- Located throughout the world and in the United states; common in Southeastern, mid-Atlantic, and Central states
- Fungus found in soil and other areas associated with bat guano or bird droppings
- Affects the lungs but may go into other organs
- Often misdiagnosed

The bats had invaded the attic of the middle school. At night, one could see thousands of bats flying around the area of the building. During the day they went into the attic and settled above one particular room. This was the room where Janie taught math. The room had a terrible stench; brown droppings from the bats streaked one wall.

Students and teachers complained, but the comment they received was, "We can't get rid of the bats." Finally, a school board member threatened to have the health department shut the school down unless something was done. The district found a way. In all, Janie had been complaining about the condition of the room for three years. Janie suffered with health problems and missed a lot of school. She had coughs and lung infections. Later, she developed kidney problems and cancer behind the sternum that could not be treated. When she died, she was tested for histoplasmosis. Tests were positive; she had the antibodies for histoplasmosis. No one had detected it, and the school district appeared not aware of the danger to the teacher and to students.

Although it is rare, it is often misdiagnosed, because people may not make the connection of being in a contaminated area or in a cave. Janie never told the doctors that she taught in the room with a bat problem. It only came out after her death.

WHAT IS HISTOPLASMOSIS?

Histoplasmosis is an infection caused by the fungus *Histoplasma capsulatum.* This organism grows as a mold in the soil or other areas, and like other molds it gives off spores. If people breathe these spores, they may get sick, usually from some type of lung infection. The area in the soil is associated with decaying bat guano or bird droppings. If these bat guano or bird droppings are in areas where new excavation is disturbing the mold, spores are released into the air. It is especially found in caves, in which cave explorers or spelunkers may disturb soil that has not been moved for years.

In 1903, efforts to build the Panama Canal were being thwarted by diseases such as yellow fever and malaria. That same year Samuel Taylor Darling (1872–1925) graduated from medical school and went to study tropical disease in the area. Walter Reed found that the mosquito carried the two main diseases, but another was causing havoc with the lungs and other body systems of the workers. In the 1930s, Darling autopsied workers who had died from the unusual lung disorder, and discovered a fungus was present in the lungs of the men. He concluded that the widespread lung and body infection was caused by spores of this fungus, which the men had breathed in.

The word "histoplasmosis" comes from the Greek terms: *histo*, meaning "tissue," *plasm*, meaning "form" or "mold," and *osis*, meaning "condition of." Although referred to as histoplasmosis, it is also known as Darling's disease.

The mold grows in the soil or in litter near where birds or bats have been. The litter around bird roosts, chicken houses, caves, or an area harboring bats may harbor the mold. Molds reproduce by forming mycelia that have spores on the end. These spores break off and go into the air. If inhaled by a human, at 37°C, it morphs into a yeast and finds its way into the alveoli or air sacs of the lungs. In the lungs, it is attacked by macrophages, a type of antibody. Macrophages travel in the lymphatic system to other organs of the body. If the patient has a strong immune system, the invaders will be calcified, but if the person has some other type of condition that has compromised the immune system, it will spread to the other organs and infect them. However, the lungs can develop a chronic disease.

WHAT ARE THE SIGNS AND SYMPTOMS?

Some people may have no symptoms; others may have symptoms that resemble many other diseases: fever, chills, cough, chest pain that gets worse when breathing, joint pain, mouth sores, and red bumps on the skin. Symptoms can begin within three to 17 days after exposure, with an average of 12 to 14 days. The acute phase is like flu with respiratory infection, which goes away after several days.

For others, the infection may become chronic. The person has chest pain and shortness of breath, cough with spitting up blood, and fever and sweating. In addition, it may spread throughout the body and affect the lining around the heart or pericardium and present headache and neck stiffness form swelling in the meninges covering the brain and spinal cord.

HOW IS IT DIAGNOSED?

The doctor may order a biopsy of the lung, skin, liver, or bone marrow, as well as blood and urine tests. A sputum test may provide the clearest results but can take over 6 weeks to be processed. Other tests may include X-ray of chest, chest CT (computed tomography) scan, bronchosopy, and a spinal tap to look for signs of infection.

WHAT IS THE TREATMENT?

If the person has a strong immune system, the condition may go away without any treatment. Antifungal medications such as amphotericin B followed by oral itraconazole or ketoconazole are usual treatments. However, these medications may cause side effects. In severe cases, treatment may last up to a year.

For Further Information

Daniel, Thomas M., and Gerald L. Baum. *Drama and Discovery: The Story of Histoplasmosis.* Santa Barbara, CA: Praeger, 2002.

Jellyfish Sting: Just When You Thought It Was Safe to Go Back in the Water

- Jellyfish are free-swimming marine animals that move with a large umbrella-like float and long tentacles
- Tentacles are used for catching food by injecting poison into prey
- Stings to humans are painful and can be life-threatening
- Can usually be self-treated

On the Atlantic coast off Riviera Beach, Florida, a 67-year-old local woman was swimming in waist-deep water. Although she weighed nearly 200 pounds and was a borderline diabetic, she was a good swimmer and was basically healthy. She jumped out of the water with something wrapped around her left leg. It had a blue float and long tentacles. Lifeguards went into action and sprayed the tentacles with a mixture containing papain and peeled them off with paper towels. When the ambulance arrived, she had stopped breathing, lost consciousness, and after five days on a ventilator, died. She had had an encounter with a Portuguese man-o-war (*Physalia physalis*). The beaches of Florida at certain times of the year are closed because of the presence of many of these animals.

Going to the beach is a part of summer recreation for many people, but individuals do need to be aware that there are animals in the sea that may cause pain, suffering, or even death. Jellyfish encounters are rare, but get lots of media attention when they do occur.

WHAT IS A JELLYFISH?

Actually, what people see is not just one jellyfish, but a collection of animals that live as a colony. Some of the animals make up the gas-filled, blue float. Others are designated for reproduction, while others maintain the stinging tentacles. As one animal, it floats on the surface and is usually found in large groups called navies. When one is sighted, the beach patrol assumes other members of its navy are around. The warnings go up, and are publicized in the media.

Like all jellyfish, these animals are predators. They hunt for their prey using their long tentacles that have at the end structures called nematocysts, which are specialized stinging structures to kill fish and other food. When a human encounters one of these animals, pressure builds up inside the nematocyst, and it bursts. A lance inside the nematocyst pierces the person's skin, and venom flows into it. The body reacts to the sting of the jellyfish because of the toxin that is released with the sting. Just being touched by a jelly fish can be painful, and even beached and dying animals can still sting.

Throughout the world there are several species of jellyfish. Australia has the most deadly jellyfish. One of these deadly animals is the Portuguese man-o-war or Bluebottle. Another jellyfish that is quite small is called the sea wasp or box jellyfish. This box jellyfish is also known as the infamous toxic Irukandji jellyfish, which is very small, but almost always deadly. Their stinging cells are triggered not by pressure, but by chemicals on the skin of their prey. The Australians have found an ingenious way to protect themselves: wear panty hose. The stingers cannot get to the skin.

WHAT ARE THE SIGNS AND SYMPTOMS?

Although humans seldom die from the stings, they are extremely painful. The pain is almost immediate. Long red lines and welts appear, which resemble a string of beads. The person often will have headache, vomiting, and abdominal pain. Some of the pain may last for hours.

HOW IS IT DIAGNOSED?

Many people who go to the beach do not go for diagnosis of a small jellyfish sting. Frequent beachgoers takes small vials of papain, such as papain meat tenderizer, which helps alleviate the sting. However, if the person emerges from the water with obvious stings, lifeguards are trained to help in this situation. Those with serious stings will be sent to the emergency room.

WHAT IS THE TREATMENT?

One of the first actions to take to help a person who has been stung is to make sure that the rescuer is protected. Rescuers wear protective clothing such as pantyhose, wet suits, or full body stingproof suits. The person must be taken out of the water. The second action is to deactivate the venom. The best procedure is to wash with the area with salt water to deactivate the stinging cells.

A box jellyfish must be treated a little differently. The tentacles should be washed with vinegar. Do not use tap water or fresh water. Baking soda may also deactivate the cells. To decontaminate and remove tentacles, rinse the area with vinegar for at least 30 seconds. Next, soak the area in hot water for at least 20 minutes. Cold packs can be used if water is not available. Calling for medical attention is essential for this sting. An antivenom may be available for box jellyfish stings.

For those stung in the Atlantic, vinegar is not recommended, and may actually make the symptoms worse. Recommended is a hot rinse and the anesthesia lidocaine applied to the area.

The next procedure is to treat discomfort using a mild hydrocortisone or oral antihistamine to relieve itching and swelling. As a follow up, use ice packs and over-the-counter pain relievers for welts. If the reaction is severe, the person may be in the hospital for several days.

For Further Information

Gershwin, Lisa-ann. *Stung!: On Jellyfish Blooms and the Future of the Ocean.* Chicago: University of Chicago Press, 2014.

Pellagra: Disease of the 4Ds

- Found mostly in developing countries where corn is the major source of food
- Sporadic cases occur in people with long-term alcoholism, people with anoxia, those who take drugs, and patients with malabsorption disorders
- Results from the lack of vitamin B_3 (niacin) or tryptophan in the diet
- Disease of four Ds: diarrhea, dermatitis, dementia, death

Pellagra is a disease that results from lack of vitamin B_3 (niacin) or tryptophan in the diet. In areas where corn and corn products are major source of food, there are more cases. It is a serious disease with results often expressed as the 4 D's: diarrhea, dermatitis, dementia, and death. Although it is rare among those who eat well-rounded diets, it is sometimes seen in immigrants, especially those from Haiti and South American countries. Many doctors who have not seen these cases before do not recognize the disease.

WHAT IS PELLAGRA?

Pellagra is a disease caused by severe vitamin B$_3$ (niacin) deficiency. The body requires niacin for many of its functions. It is required for certain body enzymes to function. The vitamin is found in animal proteins, such as chicken, beef, fish, and liver. It is also in many fruits and vegetables, such as avocado, dates, passion fruit, mushrooms, broccoli, and asparagus. It can also be made in the body from tryptophan, an essential amino acid. However, tryptophan itself is not made in the body, so the individual must get it from their diet. Such foods as chicken, turkey, eggs, sunflower seeds, pumpkin seeds, peanuts, and soy beans are sources of tryptophan. In addition, a deficiency of the amino acid lysine can lead to the condition.

Throughout history, pellagra has been a scourge of poor peasants and those whose nutrition was sub-par. In Italy, a terrible endemic condition called Hiob disease, with similar symptoms to pellagra, was referred to as the stigmata of Saint Francis of Assisi. An Italian, Francesco Frapoli referred to it as *vulgo pelagrain* from two Italian words: *pella* meaning "skin" and *agra* meaning "sour." The first case of pellagra that was described in a medical journal was found in Oviedo, Asturias, an area in northeastern Spain. In 1762, Gaspar Casal (1681–1759) noted that many of the very poor peasants had a terrible red and glossy rash on the body, hands, and feet. He called it *mal de la rose.* He then noted lesions around the neck, which were later dubbed the "Casal necklace." He was the first to make the connection between the symptoms of the condition and people who ate mostly corn or maize, and little meat, to pellagra.

In the American South, pellagra became an epidemic around the end of the 19th century. A. J. Bollet wrote about U.S. epidemics of pellagra in a 1992 edition of *The Yale Journal of Biology and Medicine,* in which he found that more than 3 million Americans had had pellagra, and that more than 100,000 had died. In his study, he told of how pellagra was stopped in the United States. In 1915 Dr. Joseph Goldberger (1874–1929) was assigned by the Public Health Service to study pellagra, and established that a small amount of brewer's yeast should be added to the diet. Goldberger's discovery was a landmark event in the history of American medicine.

Still, Goldberger did not find the actual cause. In 1937, Conrad Elvehjem (1901–1962) of Madison, Wisconsin used niacin to cure a group of dogs with black tongue disease. Later in 1938, Drs. Tom Spies, Marion Blankenship, and Clark Cooper found that niacin cures pellagra in humans.

Lack of niacin in the diet causes pellagra. For over two centuries, pellagra was endemic among areas in Europe whose people mostly ate a diet of mostly corn. Many doctors of the time proposed that maize had some toxic substance, or was the carrier of the disease. Maize was even banned in France in the early 19th century. However, it was found that corn raised by the natives of the New World did not seem to be connected with pellagra. The Native Americans used a special process to grind the corn, which did not appear to deplete the supply of niacin.

Pellagra today is still seen in certain areas of developing countries, such as North Korea, Africa, Indonesia, and China, where corn or corn products are the main source of food. In addition, other medical conditions can cause pellagra. People who are on fad diets, or individuals with anorexia nervosa may develop the symptoms. Other diseases include chronic alcohol abuse, carcinoid syndrome, and other vitamin B deficiencies. Some medications, such as isoniazid, used to treat tuberculosis, may evoke the syndrome. In addition, a genetic condition called Hartnup disease, in which the amino acids such as tryptophan are not absorbed in the gastrointestinal (GI) tract, may also cause the disorder.

WHAT ARE THE SIGNS AND SYMPTOMS?

The symptoms of pellagra are referred to as the four Ds: diarrhea, dermatitis, dementia, and death.

- **Diarrhea.** The first symptoms of the disease begin in the GI tract; pellagra begins in the stomach, but then attacks the entire lining of the GI tract. Sores in the mouth develop, along with nausea, vomiting, and diarrhea. A smooth glossy tongue may develop.
- **Dermatitis.** At first, a rash develops that resembles sunburn. Then the rash becomes darker with dark pigmentation, blisters, and skin sloughing off on the face, arms, and neck. The rash may both itch and burn, and later on, the person may become disfigured. The person may lose his or her hair. Swelling or edema is common.
- **Dementia.** The person may develop sensitivity to bright light and exhibit other emotional disturbances, such as aggression, mental confusion, hallucinations, and depression. This is usually in the later stages of the disease.
- **Death.** If the person is not treated, death is inevitable within a few years.

HOW IS IT DIAGNOSED?

Diagnosis of this condition is difficult for doctors in the Western world, because it has not been seen in contemporary times except in textbooks. If a person presented with the symptoms now, the doctor probably would not suspect pellagra. However, a recent report from a Miami hospital indicated that doctors have seen cases among immigrants, especially from Haiti.

WHAT IS THE TREATMENT?

If left untreated, the disease can kill within three to five years. The treatment is to prescribe nicotinamide, which has a similar structure to niacin but does not have the side effects of large doses of niacin itself, which can cause flushing and nausea. Most doctors recommend taking a dally multivitamin with a high protein diet for more complete healing. Pellagra, in the past 80 years, has not been seen often in the United States.

For Further Information

Jarrow, Gail. *Red Madness: How a Medical Mystery Changed What We Eat*. Honesville, PA: Calkins Creek, 2014.

Pneumoconiosis: Inhaling Dust

- An occupational disease caused by inhaling dust in the work environment of any one of several jobs
- Usually takes 20 to 30 years to develop
- About 125,000 deaths a year result from pneumoconiosis
- Common forms are silicosis, from breathing silicon particles, and black lung disease, from breathing coal dust

Coal played a major part in the booming economies of the Industrial Revolution. Extracted from the earth using deep shaft mines, coal remains a significant contributor to modern life by being a part of the process to generate electricity, produce steel, manufacture cement, and provide fuel. However, when the workers in these mines began to have breathing problems, a struggle ensued to determine that the disorder was the result of the occupation. In 1969, Congressman Ken Heckler from West Virginia led the fight to recognize that black lung was caused by coal dust. Soon, not only mining coal but many other occupations were found to damage the lungs.

WHAT IS PNEUMOCONIOSIS?

Pneumoconiosis is a chronic occupational disease of people who work in areas where small particles of dust are breathed in. The particles are microscopic about 1/5000 of an inch across, or perhaps even smaller. Because they are so tiny, they can reach the deepest part of the lungs and stay there. They cannot be removed.

Let's look briefly the way one breathes normally. When one breathes in, air with fresh oxygen passes from the nose and mouth to the trachea or windpipe that is located in the throat. The trachea then branches into two sections called the bronchi.

The bronchi branch off into smaller tubes called the bronchioles. The bronchioles branch into smaller and smaller structures until they end at the alveoli or air sacs, which are like tiny balloons. The thin membrane of the air sacs come in close contact with the circulating blood, and exchange carbon dioxide, the waste product from the body cells, for fresh, breathed-in oxygen that will nourish the cells. Carbon dioxide is then exhaled through a reverse path. Tiny hairs, called cilia, line the respiratory tract and filter dust particles and bacteria as air comes in.

However, if the air is laden with very small particles, such as coal dust, the normal cleansing process is overwhelmed, and over the years, enough of the tiny dust particles reach the air sacs in the lungs and begin to accumulate. The body starts to react against the particles by thickening and scarring. This process is called fibrosis. The little air sacs slowly lose their function, as more and more particles are deposited in the air sacs and surrounding tissues, and the body's cells cannot get the oxygen that they need.

The word "pneumoconiosis" comes from Greek words *pneumo,* meaning "lung," *coni,* meaning "dust," and *osis,* meaning "condition of." Pneumoconiosis comes in many types, depending on the kind of dust breathed in. Following is a list of diseases caused by breathing in small dust particles:

- **Silicosis.** This condition, also known as "Potter's Rot," is caused when a worker inhales anything containing silica, one of the most abundant minerals on Earth. People working with a number of materials such as sandstone, marble, flint, slate, soil, drilling, plaster, and sand may breathe in this dust. These workers are usually involved in breaking up, crushing, cutting, or sandblasting. The condition is developed over a period of 20 years or more, and the workers may not be aware that they have it until serious symptoms appear. However, there is a form that can develop after intense exposure to silicon over short periods of time.
- **Coalworker's lung.** This condition is also known as black lung, miner's lung, or anthracosis. This lung disease is caused by inhaling coal mine dust. According to the National Institute for Occupational Safety and Health (NIOSH), about one in 20 miners develop this condition. The awareness of this as a condition prompted the Federal Coal Mine Health and Safety Act of 1969. It also led to awareness of other occupational hazards.
- **Asbestosis.** Asbestos is an insulating material that is used in many areas of the building industry. It is second to silicosis in severity. A cancerous condition of the lining of the respiratory tract called mesothelioma can result from breathing asbestos.
- **Berylliosis.** Beryllium is an element used in the manufacture of fluorescent lamps. Not only can the workers get this condition from the dust, but if they bring any of the dust into their homes by having it on their clothing, family members can also get it.

- **Talcosis.** Talc is a fine substance used in many powders, and is really a type of silicosis.
- **Bauxite fibrosis.** Bauxite is the ore that processed aluminum comes from.
- **Siderosis.** This condition results from breathing in iron dust; another condition called silicosiderosis comes from dust in which silica and iron are mixed.
- **Stannosis.** This condition arises from those who work in mines where tin oxide is present.
- **Labrador lung.** This condition is found among miners in Labrador, Canada, who breathe dust mixed with iron, silica, and anthophyllite, a type of asbestos.
- **Breathing in any kind of fine dust.** These dusts include barium, graphite (used in pencil lead), mica, or others. One case was reported regarding some chefs who suffered a lung disorder from breathing in dust from cocoa when making chocolate goodies.

The types of occupations that should be watched include the following: abrasives manufacturing, asbestos removal, ceramics workers, fabric manufacturing, foundry workers, mining, quarrying, road and building construction, sand blasting, stone cutting, and iron workers. One unexpected condition may affect popcorn workers who get a lung disease from the dust and dactyl emissions from the butter flavoring used in microwave popcorn production.

WHAT ARE THE SIGNS AND SYMPTOMS?

Major signs are shortness of breath, exertion after a short amount of exercise, and coughing. In addition, each one of the conditions may have specific symptoms. For example, people with silicosis may experience blue-tinged skin, chest pain, heart disease, weight loss, and severe respiratory problems.

HOW IS IT DIAGNOSED?

Typically, the condition is found in an X-ray, although now digital imaging is used increasingly. The film will be patchy with cloudiness in the spaces between the alveoli, called the interstitial spaces.

WHAT IS THE TREATMENT?

Because the condition is developed over a long period of time, people may not be aware until symptoms become extremely serious. At this stage, there is no cure. Prevention is now the main initiative. As part of the 1969 Federal Coal Mine Health and Safety Act, miners are X-rayed every couple of years. If there is evidence of black lung, they are offered a transfer to a job outside the mine.

For Further Information

Kee, Kenneth. *A Simple Guide to Pneumoconiosis, Treatment and Related Diseases.* Printed by Amazon Digital Services, 2014.

Poison Ivy: Leaves of Three—Let Them Be

- About 70 percent of people are susceptible to exposure to the plants called poison ivy, oak, or sumac
- Over 350,000 people each year affected in the United States
- Rash is not spread from one person to another
- Can be serious if extensive

There is an old rhyme: "Leaves of three, let them be." It may help introduce the idea that a plant may be poisonous. But this does not tell the whole story. The rhyme applies to poison ivy and poison oak, but other nonharmful plants, such as blackberry or raspberry, have a similar pattern of leaf arrangement. So what is this plant that people may think they know about, when some of its effects are still unknown? Poison ivy is a general term.

WHAT IS THE POISON PLANT FAMILY?

The poison plant family *Toxicodendron radicans* has a solid reputation for being a problem, but few really know the plant and the consequences of contact with it. The plant itself, with its bright shiny leaves that turn crimson in the fall, is quite pretty. But the itching, irritation, and painful rash caused by contact with the oil called urushiol (pronounced yoo-ROO-shee-all) is not pleasant.

Actually, this plant is not a true ivy, but simply a variety of plant that can appear as a vine, shrub, or climbing vine that grows on trees or other supports. The plant grows throughout North America, Canada, and all areas except major desert areas. It is even spread as far as Russia and China.

There are four main characteristics of the plant:

- Cluster of three leaflets
- Alternate leaf arrangement
- Lack of thorns
- Each group of three leaflets has its own stem that then connects to the main vine

Sometimes the plant is difficult to recognize during different seasons, but regardless, all parts of the plant—the stem, leaves, and roots, have the oil and can cause a rash. The oil can be carried on clothing, pet hair, tools, or anything that has touched the leaves. The oil can remain active for years.

If the leaves or vines are burned, people can get poisoning from inhaling the smoke or from getting smoke in their eyes.

Contact with the oil produces contact dermatitis, the result of the interaction of the oil on the skin. The epidermis, which is the outer layer of the skin, is the mainstay of the immune system. Here, the Langerhans cells form the first line of defense against assaults from the environment. The epidermis protects the body from all kinds of insults, including the plant known as poison ivy.

Here is what happens: urushiol is a chemical within the sap of the ivy plants, and when it comes near the skin, it immediately binds to it. Once on the skin, the T-lymphocytes in the skin recognize it as a foreign invader, called an antigen. The T-cells send out signals called cytokines, telling the immune system to get to work and pump up the volume of white blood cells. T-cells direct these white blood cells to turn into macrophages, which might be thought as Super Pac-Men sent out to engulf the foreign substance urushiol. In fighting the oily urushiol, normal tissue is inflamed, and annoying dermatitis happens.

This simple leaf affects more than 350,000 people in the United States each year. There is a wide range of reactions and sensitivities to it. Some people may be especially sensitive to the blistering and oozing fluid that occurs when blood vessels develop gaps and leak fluid through the skin. About 25 percent of people exposed have no allergic reaction; however there are some that react violently, and go into a condition known as anaphylactic shock, in which breathing may stop.

WHAT ARE THE SIGNS AND SYMPTOMS?

Generally, the person who is allergic to the plant will first develop red streaks or general redness where the plant oil touched. Small bumps may then break out. The bumps will have blisters that may break and leak fluid. Contrary to popular thought, it is not the fluid that spreads the rash, and it is not contagious. The rash may take a few days to form, but it will only occur in the areas that the plant touched. The rash may last from 10 days to three weeks, but may persist up to six weeks in some cases.

Some people who are very allergic to the oil may have swelling of the face, mouth, neck, or genitals. Eyelids may close. These people may also have widespread blisters that ooze lots of fluid. They are advised to see a physician immediately because they are in danger of going into anaphylactic shock.

HOW IS IT DIAGNOSED?

People who have been in the outdoors where the plants are growing may know that the itch and mild rash is poison ivy. They may self-treat with over-the-counter creams such as Ivy-Dry. However, those who have more extensive exposure may need to go to the emergency room for diagnosis and additional treatment.

WHAT IS THE TREATMENT?

A mild rash can be taken care of at home. It is recommended that one immediately wash the area with lots of soap and water, then wash all clothes or tools that have come in contact with the plant. Use a cool wet cloth, or soak the area in cool water. Use some type of lotion, such as calamine lotion, or some specialty treatments that are available over-the-counter at the drug store. It is exceedingly important not to scratch the area, because that can cause infection. According to the Centers for Disease Control and Prevention (CDC), certain medicines are *not* recommended for use because they can cause other problems including antihistamines such as Benadryl, benzocaine (lanacane), or antibiotics containing neomycin (neosporin) applied to the skin.

If the person develops serious symptoms, it is important to see a physician at once. If he or she has a problem breathing or swallowing, or if the rash is on most of the body, they must go to the emergency room.

Prevention is worth more than the cure. Cover all body parts when working in an area where there is poison ivy. There are some products called ivy blockers that help prevent the skin from absorbing the oil. However, the best strategy is to be able to recognize the plant and avoid it if possible.

For Further Information

Hauser, Susan Carol. *Field Guide to Poison Ivy, Poison Oak, and Poison Sumac: Prevention and Remedies.* Guilford, CT: Falcon Guides, 2008.

Prune Belly Syndrome: "Little Buddha"

- Also known as Eagle-Barrett syndrome; triad syndrome; urethral obstruction malformation sequence; Obrinsky syndrome
- Affects about 1 per 30,000 to 40,000 births; 97 percent are males
- Child is born with a large stomach that appears similar to pictures of the Buddha
- Mortality is about 20 percent

Have you ever left your hands in water for a long period of time, then when you took them out, they looked wrinkled and puffy like the skin of a prune? That is what happens in prune belly syndrome. Children are born with large, wrinkled, distended bellies.

Children born with large distended stomachs have puzzled doctors for many years. In 1839 a German physician, F. Frölich, reported about children who were born with distended wrinkled stomachs and other kidney and bladder problems. The Canadian doctor William Osler (1849–1919) called the condition prune belly syndrome. In the 1950s, two doctors, J. F. Eagle and G. S. Barrett, studied nine cases of children who had prune belly and genitourinary problems. Sometimes, the disorder is called Eagle-Barrett syndrome. Another doctor, W. Obrinsky, at about the same time also wrote about the condition; it is sometimes called by his name. However, the support foundation the Prune Belly Syndrome Network calls it "prune belly syndrome."

WHAT IS PRUNE BELLY SYNDROME?

Prune belly syndrome (PBS) is a birth defect in which the child shows several abnormal conditions. It is basically present before birth, as a result of loss of the mother's amniotic fluid. What causes this is unknown. When the child is born, the abdominal region looks shriveled like a prune, hence the name prune belly syndrome. Although the cause is still debatable, prune belly syndrome is included in the environmental section of unusual disorders, because it is the conditions that exist in the mother's uterus—the surroundings of the child—that cause the disorder.

The problem actually begins in pregnancy. The mother may not have enough amniotic fluid, a condition called oligohydramnios. Most scientists agree that prune belly is not a genetic disease, but one that occurs during embryonic development. During the sixth through the 10th weeks of a pregnancy, the fetus is very susceptible to noxious events. This is the time when the mesodermal layer, which relates to the gastrointestinal development and other systems in the area, is forming. The fetus is very susceptible to noxious occurrences, such as the mother's drug or alcohol use or other outside influence. In the uterus, the baby's abdomen swells with fluid. The cause can usually be traced to a urinary tract abnormality. At birth, the fluid disappears, leaving the prune appearance. Weakness in the abdominal muscles emphasizes the look. The actual cause is still unknown and debatable.

WHAT ARE THE SIGNS AND SYMPTOMS?

The first symptom is the appearance of the wrinkled abdomen and the weak abdominal muscles. The children have a large stomach, as seen in images of the Buddha, and are sometimes referred to as a "Little Buddha." The weak abdominal muscles cause constipation and other gastrointestinal problems. Urinary infections and two undescended testicles are common genitourinary problems. In addition, the child may have heart, bone, and muscle problems. Coughing may be difficult because of increased lung secretions. As the child gets older, developmental delays in sitting and walking can occur.

Prune belly is a life-threatening condition. Many infants are stillborn or die within days. Some of the children who do survive have a normal life, but others continue to have problems throughout life.

HOW IS IT DIAGNOSED?

A physician using ultrasound can diagnose the syndrome before birth. One indicator is that the child will have a very large abdominal region resembling that of an obese person. Other abnormalities can be detected before birth. Specialists can then be on hand at birth, to treat certain abnormal conditions that may occur. When the baby is born, the abdominal muscles shrink, leaving the wrinkled or prune-like appearance.

WHAT IS THE TREATMENT?

Doctors disagree on the treatment. Some physicians may recommend a conservative wait-and-see approach, while others may want to begin aggressive therapy within a week or so after birth. Infections are inevitable. Even with aggressive treatment, there may still be complications from kidneys or bladder, which may result in the child's going on dialysis or requiring a kidney transplant.

For Further Information
Prune Belly Syndrome Network. http://prunebelly.org/.

Solenopsis invicta: **Ants of Fire**

- An ant that invaded from South America and is now in all the southern United States
- Sting can cause itching, burning blisters on the skin
- Can cause anaphylactic shock in some people
- Only way of controlling is by chemical controls

Deborah, 26, had Type I diabetes from birth. She had not taken care of herself, and had spent her teen and young adult years partying and drinking. At about 25, she lost her eyesight and developed diabetic neuropathy. She was eventually confined to a wheelchair, because of the inability to walk. One day her mother put her outside so she could feel the warm Florida sunshine. Her mother was not aware that Deborah's chair was placed on a bed of fire ants. Because Deborah had no feeling in her feet or legs, the ants swarmed on her and covered her body, inflicting painful bites that she was not aware of until it was too late. Her body was by then in anaphylactic shock. She died, a victim of the fire ant, *Solenopsis invicta*.

Although the *Solenopsis invicta* is found primarily in the southern United States and certain other countries, it is important for tourists and travelers to these regions to be aware of this red fire ant.

WHAT IS *SOLENOPSIS INVICTA*?

Solenopsis invicta is commonly called the red imported fire ant, or RIFA. Like other ants, the species are social insects that live together in colonies. The RIFA is not native to North America, but has its original home in the plains of Paraguay in South America. Between 1933 and 1945, the ant found its way to the United States in cargo brought in through the port of Mobile, Alabama or through Pensacola, Florida. The ant is now found throughout the lower part of the United States, from coast to coast. Also, it has been reported in the Caribbean Islands, the Far East in China, and even in Australia and New Zealand.

In their native South America, fire ant mounds are only 4 to 6 inches high, and they are controlled by other native species. But in their new land, they quickly overcame native species, and now their mounds may be as high as a foot, with tunnels that radiate out over 100 feet. They especially gain ground rapidly in fields newly cleared for homes or other uses. By 1989, as housing development spread to the southern states, the fire ant thrived in all of these states.

Every colony begins with a queen who has mated while in flight. She then drops to earth, sheds her wings, and begins by laying 10 to 20 eggs, which will develop into the care workers that become her attendants. She then will lay other eggs that will become the workers.

In 1905, H. G. Wells wrote a short story called the "Empire of the Ants," a terror tale of a Brazilian sea captain who is ordered to go to the upper Amazon to combat a species of ants with enhanced intelligence that is taking over the area. The captain finds entire villages destroyed by the ants, and after trying to kill them with firearms, decides to return downstream to warn everyone. A 1977 movie with the same title was also made.

Every year, between 30 to 60 percent of people living in the areas where the fire ants have colonies experience their stings. This ant operates differently from other ants, and from bees that sting. The fire ant grabs the skin with its jaws and then arches its back and inserts venom through its stinger. If holding on long enough, it will rotate around and keep injecting the venom into adjacent areas, so that a whole circle full of stings is visible. This ant both bites and stings.

The venom is also toxic to the nervous system. The person may go into anaphylactic shock. First the person feels faint, then feels tightness in the chest and throat. The blood pressure drops, and if the person is not seen immediately with some type of intervention, he or she may die. In extra-sensitive people, only one or two stings may evoke a reaction.

The venom itself is a solution of alkaloid compounds. These chemicals have a direct effect on a group of cells called mast cells. Discovered by scientist Paul Ehrlich (1854–1915), mast cells live both in the tissues and circulate in the bloodstream. They are populated with a substance called histamine, which acts like tiny explosives. For example, when a mast cell in the nose hits a pollen grain from the environment, it explodes and causes a raw, runny nose and itching. If a person reacts to shellfish or mangoes, mast cells in the blood may trigger a reaction called hives. Fire ant alkaloids trigger the same release of histamine from mast cells, by causing damage to the tissues. That is why everyone who is stung develops the same kind of welts and pustules. No preexisting allergy is needed.

WHAT ARE THE SIGNS AND SYMPTOMS?

Almost everyone reacts to the bite and sting. The person feels an immediate burning and painful itching. A small welt develops that in a day or so becomes white with pus. Up to half of the people bitten will have serious local infections that necessitate surgical draining, and if the reaction is extreme, amputation.

HOW IS IT DIAGNOSED?

The burning, itching welts are a clue that the person has been bitten. Many people treat themselves with creams and lotions to stop the itch. However, if the person develops a fever or cannot breathe, he or she must go to the emergency room.

WHAT IS THE TREATMENT?

Fire ants do not appear to avoid areas covered with insecticides. For those working in gardens or outside, vigilance is essential to avoid the large mounds. The best treatment for prophylaxis is early treatment with epinephrine. If the person is known to have this reaction, a product called EpiPen is preloaded for injection. This could give protection until the paramedics arrive. Some people keep benadryl in the home in case of any reaction.

If the person is really prone to reaction, a preventive measure called immunotherapy is available. These are injections made from whole ants that are given in once or twice weekly doses.

The name "invicta" was given to them for a reason. Dr. W. F. Buren gave them that name in 1965, because they are unconquerable or invincible and almost impossible to manage.

Many methods have been used. Farmers have poured gasoline and pushed ashes, citrus peels, watermelon rinds, vinegar, and grits into fire ant mounds, and still found that nothing worked. When scientists developed chemical controls, they found that local animals were harmed; hence, in a way, trying to control the fire ant created environmental movements. Farmers in 1957 found that chlorinated heptachlor could kill the ants; this chemical mixed with soybean oil and called mirex was very effective. But soon, cattle and wildlife began to die. In 1962, the book *Silent Spring* warned about these chlorinated hydrocarbons, so they were banned in 1970.

Biological controls were also considered. Thus far, using protozoa and fungal parasites that may kill isolated ants does not work in the colonies. Researchers in Florida have studied phorid flies, a fire ant enemy that lays eggs inside the ant, which makes their heads fall off. But putting a new insect into the environment may not have the desired consequences, and they may become pests themselves.

Probably no strategy will ever completely eradicate the fire ant from the United States. They will probably always be the winners, and true to their name, are invincible. The trick is to avoid them—and to be aware of the location of their hills and nest, which the workers will aggressively defend if it is disturbed.

For Further Information

Hölldobler, Bert, and Edward O. Wilson. *The Ants*. Cambridge, MA: Belknap Press of Harvard University Press, 1990.

Stachybotrys chartarum: The Toxic Black Mold

- Black mold produces a toxin that affects people in different ways
- Must have a suitable wet material, such as materials high in cellulose, to grow and produce toxins
- Found extensively in the United States and is prevalent in areas of high humidity
- Mold must be professionally removed

The Kennedy family had built a beautiful new show home in the Dallas suburbs. When Don Kennedy, a real estate agent, began to cough and have a fever, he thought it was simply the flu, however, it did not go away. Later he began to have memory issues, and at the same time, their son began to have troubles in school; he was diagnosed with a learning disability. A friend just visiting for a short time said that he was nauseated when inside the house. It was then, after months of investigation, that they were told that the house was growing a type of mold that was causing black mold poisoning. The mold was caused by a leak in the refrigerator, and had extensively invaded the walls of the kitchen. The family had to move out of the house, but the symptoms for Don and their son remained for several years after treatment. The Kennedy family was reacting to a toxin produced by the black mold: *Stachybotrys chartarum*.

WHAT IS *STACHYBOTRYS CHARTARUM*?

*Stachybotrys chartarum i*s a greenish black fungus that grows in nature and other environments. It produces a long filament or mycelium where spores for reproduction develop. The spores fly off into the air to begin new growth. The spores have been found in grains, insulator foams, indoor air, and especially in water-damaged buildings. The mold was first reported in the 1920s in Russia, where horses and cattle that had eaten moldy hay died. Later, in the 1970s, people in Southeast Asia began dying from "Yellow Rain." The cause was traced to the mycotoxins that were aerosolized and then combined with rain in the air.

The growth appears black, shiny, and glistening, giving it a slimy look. It grows on material that has a high cellulose content, such as wicker, wood chips, cardboard boxes, paper files, the paper covering of gypsum wallboard, particleboard, and wood, when any of these materials become and remain wet. The mold requires high humidity for days and weeks to begin to grow, and takes about 48 hours of sustained wetness to begin growth. Therefore, the slow water leak in a wall creates ideal conditions. Spills from showers or bathtubs, or leaking roofs, may cause many types of molds, including *Stachybotrys*.

The toxin that is produced is known as trichothecene mycotoxin, or satratoxin. The poison can cause changes in animal and human tissues, leading to serious medical problems. Natural disasters such as Hurricane Katrina leave thousands of homes with water damage. Water damage combined with the heat and humidity that is present after a hurricane are ideal settings for mold growth.

Stachybotrys in the body creates mycotoxins that affect the biological systems. These toxins are far more deadly than pesticides or heavy metals, because the living fungi can mutate and bypass the immune system, while at the same time producing chemicals that suppress the immune system. So if the immune system is compromised in any way, or if the person has a tendency to react to other allergens, mold can pose a significant risk. In addition, the inhaled mold toxin can cross from the nose and eyes to the brain, causing neurological and behavioral problems, such as the Kennedy family experienced. Long-term exposure can lead to death. According to a public health report in Cleveland in 1994, sudden infant death syndrome (SIDS) may be linked to mold exposure.

WHAT ARE THE SIGNS AND SYMPTOMS?

Many types of mold can cause health problems, and few people have made the connection between the two. Other molds such as *Cladosporium, Penicillium*, and *Aspergillus* (common bread mold) can also cause problems. *Stachybotrys* is less common than these types, but it is not rare.

Stachybotrys poisoning can occur when someone is exposed to the mold spores that create toxins that affect the person. In 2004 the Institute of Medicine (IOM) released a study that showed this type of mold exposure was linked to upper respiratory infections. The symptoms may begin as headaches, dizziness, swollen lymph glands, chronic fatigue syndrome, runny nose, nausea, digestive issues, and eye irritation. Because these symptoms are common in many other health conditions, mold toxins are probably not the first thing to be considered. In fact, one study proposes that mold and its toxins are the sources of almost all sinus infections, but these are misdiagnosed and then mistreated. Humans with chronic exposure to *Stachybotrys* have also reported more serious conditions, including memory loss, muscle ache, hair loss, cancer, pulmonary hemorrhage, and autoimmune disease.

HOW IS IT DIAGNOSED?

Diagnosing mold poisoning presents a challenge. Knowledge regarding this condition is not something that an ordinary health care practitioner has. Physicians should have training in environmental medicine and understand the battery of tests that may be required. Tests include immune tests for autoantibodies, urine and blood testing for mycotoxins, neurological test batteries, and certain metabolic tests for thyroid hormone level. Diagnosis is imperative to get the proper treatment from a specialist. The presence of the symptoms of this poisoning may be similar to many other disorders: lack of memory, constant illness, behavior and neurological problems. But if black mold is seen growing in the house, individuals should share this with their health care provider.

WHAT IS THE TREATMENT?

If a person has been identified with the problem, he or she should immediately move out of the house and have it treated. Experts agree that all types of mold growths should be treated. Sometimes, people want to save money and try to get rid of the mold on their own. However, the spores are dangerous during the cleanup period because of the exposure while cleaning and disinfecting. The person cleaning must wear rubber gloves and be sure to wash all clothing immediately. Leaving such clothing around can provide a place for mold to grow.

If damage is extensive or is too much for the homeowner to manage, a professional mold specialist should be called. The professional cleaner will set up

---

PREVENTING BLACK MOLD

Several suggestions may help:
- Keep humidity as low as you can, which would be no higher than 50 percent.
- Use an air conditioner or dehumidifier during humid months.
- Be sure that the home has adequate ventilation, especially in kitchen and bathroom.
- Add mold inhibitors to paints.
- Clean bathrooms with mold-killing products.
- Do not carpet bathrooms.
- Remove and replace flooded carpets.

---

containments for sucking the mold out of the air with negative air pressure. They will purify the air with a HEPA filter or scrubber, and will remove parts that are affected, bag them, and use the HEPA vacuum again. The area will be cleaned with a disinfectant, then thoroughly dried.

All roof leaks, leaky windows, or pipe leaks should be fixed, or the mold will return. The area must be completely dry, because dampness can lead to additional mold growth.

Unfortunately, there is no cure or antidote for toxic black mold. The person must be removed from the contaminated environment. It may take time for the body to recover from the symptoms.

For Further Information

Progovitz, Richard F. *Black Mold: Your Health and Your Home.* Cleveland, NY: Forager Press, 2003.

Tech Neck Syndrome: A Real Pain in the Neck

- A new condition of the digital age
- Cervical aches caused by consistent use of digital devices
- May affect up to 60 percent of Americans
- Can be prevented with proper posture and device positioning

Jennifer had a constant neck pain. She went to the chiropractor, which gave her temporary relief, but the pain returned. One day she noticed that the pain returned the more she stayed hunched over her smartphone. She loved information and was on it constantly, emailing, looking at interesting blogs, or reading books from the phone. She even wrote her college term papers on the smartphone. Then she had a revelation. Hunching over the smartphone was giving her the neck pain. She was a victim of tech neck syndrome.

This disorder is a new one, spawned by the digital age. Only a few years ago, it was unknown, and still may be to a number of people who use digital devices and have been having neck problems.

WHAT IS TECH NECK SYNDROME?

At one time the term "pain in the neck" was an expression for someone or something that was extremely bothersome or annoying. Sometimes, the term was applied to sleeping "wrong," or if one woke up with a "crick" in the neck. Now it is a real term, and a syndrome that more people are experiencing as they constantly use digital devices.

It is a matter of simple biomechanics. The spine is divided into several parts: the cervical or neck area, thoracic or chest area, and lumbar or pelvic area vertebrae. When one is in a neutral or straight position, the head puts 10 to 12 pounds of manageable stress on the cervical spine in the area of the neck, and gravity is not working against it. But if one tilts the head just 15 degrees or about 2 to 3 inches downward, about 27 pounds of stress is put on the cervical spine. If the tilt of the head is 45 degrees, 49 pounds of pressure is added; at 60 degrees, 60 pounds of pressure is put upon the vertebrae in the neck. One can see how, with each successive degree bent forward, additional stress is put on the neck.

Now add all the hours that a person may spend in this hunched over position, and one can see that over time, bad things could happen. Extra stress is put on the vertebrae, leading to shearing and inflammation of the ligaments, soft tissue, and facet joints of the neck. Over time, the simple pain and headaches can become osteoarthritis and herniated discs.

WHAT ARE THE SIGNS AND SYMPTOMS?

Upper back and neck pain are the two main symptoms. The person spends hours bent over smartphones and inappropriately positioned laptops; some begin to have severe pain that does not go away. The shoulders then hunch over and become rounded, with a condition known as lordosis.

HOW IS IT DIAGNOSED?

A person with neck, shoulder, or back pain who uses the computer for hours at a time should be aware that they could develop serious problems. The person can diagnose the condition and practice good computer use. Millennials whose world revolves around technology are the ultimate victims. Some doctors, chiropractors, and physical therapists are finding more and more cases of cervical degeneration, even among elementary school kids.

WHAT IS THE TREATMENT?

People must be taught to use their smartphones so that tech neck does occur due to their working in an uncomfortable position. One chiropractor in Delray Beach, Florida who has been concerned about the necks and spines of adolescents, has started a local grassroots initiative clued "Looking Up" to remind people of all ages to keep their handheld devices at eye level. She also recommends strengthening the muscles in your body core, so that the head will not be constantly pulled forward. A key is to maintain good posture. She encourages thinking that your head being pulled straight up in the air by a hot air balloon.

For Further Information

Sloane, Matt. "'Text Neck' and Other Tech Troubles." WebMD. Last modified November 26, 2014. http://www.webmd.com/pain-management/news/20141124/text-neck.

Thalidomide Embryopathy: Birth Defects from a Drug

- Thalidomide was developed to treat morning sickness during pregnancy
- Caused 12,000 babies in 46 countries to be born with defects
- The children had defects ranging from flipper-like arms to more severe disabilities and death
- In the United States, Dr. Frances Kelsey kept the drug off the market

Terry Wiles was born in England on January 12, 1962, with severe disabilities from his mother's use of thalidomide for morning sickness. His mother abandoned him at birth to a children's home. Hazel and Len Wiles, a middle-aged childless couple, adopted him and soon began to work with this severely disabled child. Len built a series of Super-cars, a motorized wheelchair based on the forklift truck to help Terry move around. Terry learned to live an independent life and went to the local school, instead of one for students with disabilities. In 1979 the BBC presented a television program called *On Giant's Shoulders*, which told the story of Terry and his fabulous adoptive family. The family moved to New Zealand, where Terry married a nurse, and still lives there today.

WHAT IS THALIDOMIDE EMBRYOPATHY?

Thalidomide embryopathy occurs when a mother takes the drug thalidomide during her pregnancy. There are two types of embryopathies—primary, which is traced to a genetic problem, and secondary, which occurs when an outside factor is present. Thalidomide embryopathy is an example of a secondary agent.

A secondary embryopathy is a birth defect that occurs when the child is developing during pregnancy. The embryo is developing normally until exposed to the agent. The agent could be drugs and medicines, environmental chemicals, radiation, infections, or some metabolic imbalance that the mother may possess. These agents are called teratogenic factors. "Teratogenic" arises from the Greek roots *teratos*, meaning "monster," and *gen*, meaning "give rise to." The word "noxae" is used to describe the harmful agents that result in a disabled condition. In the case of thalidomide, the teratogenic drug was the noxae that gave rise to problems when the drug was taken at a particular stage of development.

Following are the stages of development of the offspring:

- **Weeks 1-2 or first 14 days:** If exposed during this time, an abnormality does not generally result
- **Third to eighth week:** The embryo is extremely vulnerable, because during these weeks organs begin to form, and many biochemical reactions are taking place. Exposure during these days can cause issues with the body part that is developing at that stage.
- **Fetal period begins at nine weeks:** Sensitivity is greatly reduced, because most organs are formed. The one exception is the cerebral cortex, the thinking part of the brain.

WHAT ARE THE SIGNS AND SYMPTOMS?

In 1956 a German pharmaceutical company called Chemie Grünenthal developed thalidomide and marketed it for respiratory infections. They also believed it was a wonder drug for morning sickness, insomnia, coughs, colds, and headaches, and aggressively marketed it as Contergan(r). At the time, testing of drugs was not as tightly controlled, and thousands of pregnant women took the drug because it was considered safe. The drug had only been tested on rodents.

However, soon babies were born with some unusual birth defects. The most common defect was malformation of the arms and limbs, but there were also some children with hearing impairments, deafness, blindness and internal injuries of the heart, kidneys, and uterus. The children with deformed or flapper-like limbs were said to have phocomelia. An Australian researcher made the connection between thalidomide and the defects. It is believed that only one pill of the powerful drug can cause developmental disorders, depending upon the phase of embryonic development.

At the beginning of 1960, about 12,000 children in 48 countries were born with thalidomide-related injuries. In November 1961, the West German Republic took it off the market. Other countries soon followed.

HOW IS IT DIAGNOSED?

The presence of the missing limbs or body parts at birth is enough for the physician to warrant a diagnosis. Diagnosis must ascertain the seriousness of the disability.

In 1960 Dr. Frances Kelsey had become the administrator for the United States Food and Drug Administration (FDA). At the time she was only one of seven full-time people working at the FDA. Her first assignment was to review the application by a pharmaceutical firm named Richardson Merrill for a drug named thalidomide. Over 20 countries had approved it for several uses, including morning sickness for pregnant women. However, she was concerned about a study from Britain that documented severe side effects on the nervous system, and withheld approval.

The drug company was not happy and put enormous pressure on her to approve the drug. She resisted. When the news of all the children born with deformities was revealed, Kelsey was hailed as a heroine. Her determination and public outcry

---

RECENT USES FOR THALIDOMIDE

Thalidomide has a checkered history; however, it has been shown to be effective in treating other diseases, and may be making a comeback. In 1985 the World Health Organization approved thalidomide again, and it is being used in over 50 countries, mostly for the treatment of leprosy in developing countries. Some organizations are concerned, because there is information about a number of children being born with the same disabilities in leper colonies in Brazil. Without proper management, including targeting people with specific conditions for treatment, another catastrophe could happen.

Following are some other uses in which thalidomide has been shown effective:

- Multiple myeloma
- Inflammatory diseases that affect the skin, such as cutaneous lupus and Behcet's disease
- HIV-related mouth and throat ulcers
- HIV-related weight loss and body wasting
- Cancers, especially bone marrow cancers, such as leukemia and myelofibrosis
- Other cancers

Some groups are very concerned about the return of thalidomide, saying that without rigid dispensing, it will fall into the wrong hands, and no one will be held responsible.

against the drug led to the 1962 Kefauver Harris Amendment to the Federal Food, Drug, and Cosmetic Act, which required companies to show the safety and effectiveness of new drugs before approval.

WHAT IS THE TREATMENT?

Depending on the area that was affected by the drug, interventions will take place. The National Health Systems of the countries with thalidomide victims have paid for prosthetic limbs and other treatments.

For Further Information

Knightley, Phillip, and Harold Evans. *Suffer The Children: The Story of Thalidomide*. New York: The Viking Press, 1979.

Stephens, Trent, and Rock Brynner. *Dark Remedy: The Impact of Thalidomide and Its Revival as a Vital Medicine*. New York: Perseus Books, 2001.

Trench Foot: A Result of Warfare

- Also known as immersion foot syndrome
- Common during the trench warfare of World War I
- Results from exposure to cold, wet, and unsanitary conditions
- If not treated, gangrene may lead to amputation

Trench warfare is a form of land fighting in which the soldiers dig trenches to protect themselves from their enemies' small arms fire and artillery. Soldiers from different countries constructed elaborate trenches and dugouts, opposing each other along a front. It was especially used during World War I. Soldiers stood for hours in waterlogged trenches with boots that were not waterproof. Their boots and socks became wet, and the exposure caused their feet to turn red or blue and to become infected. It is estimated that during the winter of 1914–1915, over 20,000 British soldiers had trench foot.

WHAT IS TRENCH FOOT?

Trench foot is a condition caused when the feet are exposed for long periods of time to damp, unsanitary, and cold conditions. It is different from frostbite, in that the weather does not have to be freezing. The soldiers stand for long hours in trenches that have standing water. The water penetrates their boots and socks. Over a number of hours, the feet become soaked, causing them to become numb and cold.

Although trench foot received notoriety during World War I, it was first seen in Napoleon's army in 1812. The French army was retreating from the Russian army. A French army surgeon Dominique Jean Larrey (1766–1842), an important innovator in battlefield medicine, first described the condition and worked to improve conditions that would prevent it.

Life in the trenches is described as living in mud and water. Trench warfare was also used in World War II and in Vietnam. The same foot condition in Vietnam was called "jungle rot." More recently, trench foot made an appearance in 1982, during the Falklands War. The British Army did not ensure proper protection for the cold and wet conditions. In addition, it may also appear when civilians go to certain events where they stand a long time in wet and muddy places. In 1998, 2007, and 2013, people going to music festivals such as those in Leeds developed trench foot.

Wet conditions for a prolonged period of time set the stage for the growth of bacteria that will then lead to tissue damage. The damage does not occur overnight, but in stages. In the first stage, blood vessels are constricted by water and moisture. No oxygen can reach the cells of the foot, because the foot is immersed in water. The feeling can be restored if the foot is taken out of the water and warmed. The second stage occurs when the foot does not get any blood flow. The blood vessels open up, and the foot begins to swell. Ulcers and blisters may form at this stage. It may take a while, but the foot can be treated with medications. The third stage involves swelling and pain. Even with treatment, there can be complications leading to the need for amputation.

WHAT ARE THE SIGNS AND SYMPTOMS?

The hours of exposure cause itchiness and rash on the skin of the feet, especially between the toes. The feet begin to tingle and swell. Blood flow to the feet is reduced, and the foot begins to turn red, then blue. The feet develop a terrible stench due to the exposure to moisture, and begin to swell. In advanced stages, blisters develop and the ulcers form that lead to gangrene.

One soldier described how his feet swelled to two or three times the normal size and then went completely dead. One could stick a bayonet in them and not feel a thing. When the swelling begins to go down, then the men may have agonizing pain. Coming with that is the realization that the foot may have to be amputated.

HOW IS IT DIAGNOSED?

When the British army realized the seriousness of this condition, they made arrangements for the men to wear oiled boots and change their socks more frequently. The implementation of "buddy" inspection helped in the diagnosis and prevention.

WHAT IS THE TREATMENT?

For treatment, the person must be removed from the water and the wet boots and socks replaced. The affected parts should be treated with warm packs or in warm water for about five minutes. Later during World War I, the soldiers discovered that they could put a board above the mud and water for standing. The army also issued three pairs of socks and treated boots with whale oil for waterproofing.

The army also implemented regular foot inspections. Soldiers would be paired with a buddy who would be responsible for another person, because if left on his own, the individual soldier might neglect doing this.

For Further Information

Bull, Stephen. *Trench: A History of Trench Warfare on the Western Front*. Oxford, UK: Osprey Publishing, 2014.

Vibrio: Take Care When Eating Oysters

- Shellfish such as oysters and clams can harbor deadly bacteria
- *Vibrio vulnificus* is the most deadly food-borne pathogen
- The risk is greatest for people who have certain diseases or compromised immune systems
- Summer is the prime time for *Vibrio*

There is an old folk saying, "Only eat shellfish [such as oysters or clams] in months with an R." This would leave out the summer months of June, July, and August. The wisdom holds true, because it is in these months that a bacterium known as *Vibrio* grows in warm waters. *Vibrio* can contaminate oysters and clams, and make some people very ill.

WHAT IS VIBRIO?

Vibrio vulnificus is a gram-negative bacterium that lives in warm seawater. The Centers for Disease Control and Prevention (CDC) first isolated this bacterium in 1964, and began documenting cases of illness and death in 1979. The bacterium grows in relationship to the warmer water temperatures, which occur normally during the summer months. The prime oyster growing regions are the Florida Gulf Coast and other coastal areas, from North Carolina to Maryland.

People may get *Vibrio* in two ways. They may consume raw or undercooked clams, finfish, or oysters, or they may get the bacterium through a cut, burn, or break in the skin when exposed to contaminated water. Adults who are healthy are at little risk, but others, such as children or those with compromised immune systems, are at risk for severe illness.

Oysters and clams are sedentary bivalve mollusks that latch onto hard surfaces and stay there. They get their food by filtering small plants and animals from the water. If *Vibrio* are in the water where the oysters feed, the bacteria are taken in and assimilated in the tissues. If people eat the oysters, they then also consume the bacteria.

WHAT ARE THE SIGNS AND SYMPTOMS?

The individual eats the raw or undercooked oysters. The bacteria multiply rapidly in the digestive tract. Healthy people can generally consume oysters without serious risk, because their immune systems will fight off the infection. However, if the person does have certain health conditions, an infection may occur. The symptoms of vibriosis, the condition caused by *Vibrio,* can occur within 24 to 48 hours, and may include sudden chills, fever, nausea, vomiting, diarrhea, shock, and skin lesions.

Some of the health conditions may be present without symptoms, so the person may not be aware of the risk. For example, drinking alcohol including beer and wine regularly may put the person at risk, though they may have no symptoms of liver disease. However, the people with the following conditions are definitely at risk: those with liver disease from hepatitis, cirrhosis, alcoholism, or cancer, people with iron overload disease or hemochromatosis, diabetes, cancer of all kinds, stomach disorders, or any illness that may compromise the body's immune system. According to the CDC, there is a greater than 50 percent mortality rate in the at-risk group.

The severe illness results from primary septicemia or blood poisoning and septic shock. If left untreated, death can occur within two days.

HOW IS IT DIAGNOSED?

The symptoms occur only after eating raw shellfish or oysters. If the person suspects that there is a connection, he or she should not self-diagnose, but seek medical attention.

WHAT IS THE TREATMENT?

The person must let the health professional know about the consumption of oysters. It is treatable with a regimen of antibiotics and supportive management.

The risk of *Vibrio* infection can be reduced by getting oysters from reputable sources, but the bacteria are not the result of pollution. Eating oysters from "clean" waters or even in reputable restaurants does not provide protection. Eating raw oysters with hot sauce or drinking alcohol does not kill the bacteria. Only heat can do that. Thorough cooking is necessary to kill the bacteria.

For Further Information

Faruque, S. M., and G. B. Nair, eds. *Vibrio cholerae: Genomics and Molecular Biology*. Norfolk, UK: Caister Academic Press, 2008.

PART IV

UNUSUAL INFECTIOUS DISEASES

WHAT YOU SHOULD KNOW ABOUT INFECTIOUS DISEASES

An infectious disease is caused by a very small organism called a microbe. The word comes from two Greek words: *micro*, meaning "small" and *bio*, meaning "life." These small organisms cannot be seen with the unaided eye; they live in a microscopic world. Following are the types of disease-causing microbes that are in this section:

- **Bacteria.** These single cell organisms are a few micrometers in length and come in basically three shapes: cocci (round), bacilli (rod-shaped), and spirilla (twisted like a corkscrew). They can be grouped by their outer cell walls, which take up or do not take up Gram stain, making them either Gram-positive or Gram-negative. It is important to note that although some bacteria can cause serious or even life-threatening diseases, many others have no health impact on humans, or actually play a beneficial role.
- **Viruses.** These organisms are much smaller than bacteria, and must have another host cell to live and reproduce in. They are basically genes made from DNA or RNA, with an outer covering. Because of their unique makeup, scientists debate whether viruses can be considered "alive" or not.
- **Fungi.** These organisms may be either unicellular or multicellular, and include yeasts and molds. Although once considered part of the plant kingdom, they are now recognized as their own unique group of organisms.
- **Protozoa.** These are unicellular organisms that do not possess a cell wall like plants or fungi and have some degree of movement. They are usually found in moist or wet environments and cover a very diverse group of organisms.

Many of the microbes that we refer to have common names, but each also has a scientific name, composed of two parts, in Latin. The first part of the name is the genus and the second part is the species name. Scientific names are always italicized. For example; *Staphylococcus aureus* is commonly referred to simply as "staph."

Many of the diseases can be spread from human-to-human contact. Others are zoonotic, meaning they are carried by animals who act as hosts and transmit the disease to humans. Still others can be transmitted by eating or drinking contaminated foods or beverages, or by coming into contact with contaminated objects and surfaces.

In the United States, the Centers for Disease Control and Prevention (CDC) is the chief national public health institute that is responsible for promoting public safety and health. It is located in Atlanta, Georgia. Some of the diseases mentioned in this section are constantly monitored by the CDC. The World Health Organization (WHO), whose headquarters is in Geneva, Switzerland, is concerned with international health and also monitors many of these diseases.

For Further Information

Infectious Diseases: MedlinePlus. National Library of Medicine. www.nlm.nih.gov /medlineplus/infectiousdiseases.html.

Moalem, Sharon. *Survival of the Sickest: The Surprising Connections between Disease and Longevity*. New York: Harper Collins, 2007.

Nagami, Pamela. *The Woman with a Worm in Her Head and Other True Stories of Infectious Disease*. New York: St. Martin's Press, 2001.

World Health Organization. Infectious Diseases. www.who.int.

Cat Scratch Disease: Carried by Furry Friends

- Also known as cat scratch fever; Teeny's Disease; inoculation lymphoreticulosis; subacute regional lymphadenitis
- Prevalence: About 22,000 new infections every year in the United States
- Cat carries bacteria that may infect humans; cats are not affected
- May clear up by itself; however, complications may result

Dorothy has a very active lifestyle. She is a busy banker, participates in community life, and stars in local tennis tournaments. When she comes home, she is greeted by her faithful cat Babe. One day while playing with Babe, she received a small scratch on the arm. Several days later, she noticed a red swollen area. The doctor said it was tennis elbow and put her arm in a sling. After several weeks of enduring the sling, the area continued to balloon, and she went back to another doctor this time. He noticed the unhealed scratch and prescribed antibiotics. The arm was soon returned to normal. This story is repeated often. The cat is not sick, but carries the bacteria that can cause infection.

WHAT IS CAT SCRATCH DISEASE?

Cat scratch disease (CSD) is an infectious condition caused by *Bartonella henselae*, a bacterium that is transmitted in the saliva of cats. Although the cats may appear healthy, they can carry the bacterium and humans can catch it through a scratch or bite, or even by petting a cat that has just licked himself. About 40 percent of cats have been identified as carriers of the bacteria sometime during their life. Kittens are more likely to be infected than older cats.

Although the infection may be benign, serious side effects may develop. Anyone who is exposed to cats can get the disease; however, serious complications may ensue in those whose immune systems are not working properly due to chemotherapy, organ transplants, or HIV/AIDS. Although *B. henselae* has been found in fleas, no evidence exists that the infected flea can pass the bacteria to humans. However, the flea may transmit the bacteria from cat to cat.

In 1889, Dr. Henri Parinaud (1844–1905), a French ophthalmologist and neurologist, saw a patient whose eye was affected by a bacterium *B. henselae* and who had symptoms similar to CSD as it is known today. The patient had been scratched by a cat. Parinaud was the first to realize that cats can carry disease. The rare, serious manifestation of CSD, Parinaud's oculoglandular syndrome, bears his name. Later in 1950, Dr. Robert Debre (1882–1978), a French pediatrician, made the connection between cats and cat scratch fever.

WHAT ARE THE SIGNS AND SYMPTOMS?

The development of the symptoms may follow this scenario. The cat scratches or nips the person. The bacteria can also be transmitted if a cat licks an area of broken skin or the white of the eye. Several days later, a small blister appears at the site of the scratch. Probably the individual does not even notice it, or ignores it.

In a few days, some other symptoms develop. The person has a fever, a headache, and generally feels ills. She or he may also notice swollen lymph nodes in the neck area and under the arms. The condition, known as lymphadenopathy, can occur anywhere lymph glands are located, such as in the arms, neck, jaw, around the ear, and in the groin.

In healthy person, the condition usually goes away on its own. However, in rare cases, which may include those with compromised immune systems or other diseases, CSD can lead to other serious symptoms. The pain may become severe, and high fever may develop. The individual must seek immediate medical care as this can develop into serious neurologic or cardiac disorders. These serious conditions include meningitis, encephalitis, seizures, or endocarditis, an inflammation of the heart. Endocarditis caused by *B. henselae* has a very high rate of mortality. The condition Parinaud's oculoglandular syndrome affects the eye. This condition is especially correlated with swelling of the lymph node near the ear.

HOW IS IT DIAGNOSED?

Although the disease is common, it is quite difficult to diagnose. Patients or doctors may confuse the symptoms with another condition. *B. hinselae*, a Gram-negative bacterium, is difficult to culture. A method called polymerase chain reaction (PCR) is the best way to test for the organism. A blood test called an immunofluorescence assay (IFA) can detect the infection, but it should be combined with other information, such as the person's medical history, other lab tests, and biopsy of the lymph nodes.

PREVENTING CSD

The Centers for Disease Control and Prevention (CDC) gives the following tips for reducing the risk of getting cat scratch disease:

- Do not play roughly with cats, especially kittens; avoid activities that may lead to scratches or bites, such as trying to play with the cat when he or she is eating.
- After playing with a cat, wash your hands thoroughly.
- Wash a bite or scratch immediately with soap and running water; put some antiseptic cream on the area.
- Do not let cats lick open wounds or sores.
- Control fleas. This is much easier now with once-a-month pills or collars.

WHAT IS THE TREATMENT?

For healthy people, the condition is not serious, and will resolve itself over a few months with or without treatment. It is not recommended that antibiotics be given to those in good health because of the potential side effects. Those with serious other diseases need prompt medical attention. Treatment with antibiotics will usually lead to recovery. For patients with complications, treatments need to be addressed on an individual basis.

For Further Information

Eldredge, Debra M. *Cat Owner's Home Veterinary Handbook*, 3rd ed. New York: Howell Book House (Wiley), 2007.

Chikungunya: A New Virus Carried by Mosquitoes

- Viral infection transmitted to humans by mosquitoes
- First appeared in the United States in 2014
- Causes fever and severe joint pain but is usually not fatal
- No specific treatment is known

Since Chikungunya virus was first diagnosed in St. Martin in the Caribbean in December 2013, it has been spreading rapidly through the Western Hemisphere. In fact, in December 2014, over 10,000 cases were reported in Puerto Rico. Cases have appeared periodically in the United States, traced to people who have traveled abroad. However, in May 2014, the first locally acquired case was confirmed in the United States. The newly confirmed case in Palm Beach County, Florida, was the first time the virus had appeared in a person who evidently acquired the infection from local mosquitoes. Health departments are concerned. However, no signs of an outbreak were associated with the case from local mosquitoes. Many people in the United States have ties to Puerto Rico.

WHAT IS CHIKUNGUNYA?

Chikungunya is a viral disease that is carried by certain mosquitoes. Two types, called *Aedes aegypti* and *Aedes albopictus*, are carriers of several diseases. The carrier *A. albopictus* is more widespread, and if any change or mutation in the viral stain occurs, it could spread the disease to many areas. Monkeys, birds, cattle, and rodents are hosts of this virus, and a human can get it from mosquitoes that act as carriers. A mosquito can bite and suck the blood of these hosts, then transmit it to a human. These two mosquitoes are different from others, in that they thrive in towns and urban areas.

The virus first appeared in Tanzania in Africa in 1952 and remained confined to Sub-Saharan Africa, the Arabian Peninsula, and Southeast Asia, except for a few travelers who might bring the virus to other parts of the world, including the United States. However, that changed in December 2013 when the first New World case appeared in St. Martin in the Caribbean. Local mosquitoes passed the infection, and soon it was in 17 different countries in the Western Hemisphere.

The word Chikungunya originated among the Makonde, a tribe that occupies areas of Tanzania and Mozambique. Chikungunya means "that which bends up," and refers to the painful contortions of the joints, bones, and muscle spasms that the disease causes.

WHAT ARE THE SIGNS AND SYMPTOMS?

The main symptoms are high fever and intense joint pain. Other symptoms include headache, muscle pain, joint swelling, nausea, vomiting, and rash. Although it is seldom lethal, the disease can be quite debilitating, especially for older people. The reactions of individuals vary. Some may have only a short period of pain and fever; others may suffer intense pain, rash, headache, and joint swelling. One person has said that you may not die, but you may wish you were dead. The condition for many is that painful.

The time from the bite of the mosquito to the beginning of symptoms ranges from two to twelve days, with the typical period being three to seven days. About 72 percent of those infected develop some of the symptoms. In addition, some people may have long-term or chronic symptoms following the acute condition. For example, in 2006 an outbreak on Reunion Island, a French territory in the Indian Ocean, revealed that over 50 percent of individuals over 45 years of age reported strong joint pain or stiffness lasting months or years. Others reported lasting effects in the eyes. Several death certificates listed Chikungunya as the cause.

HOW IS IT DIAGNOSED?

A person traveling to areas in the Caribbean or Central America should inform the health care provider if they are experiencing any unusual symptoms. In order to definitely diagnose Chikungunya, the virus can be isolated, but it takes about two weeks to do so, and this must be done under Biosafety Level 3 (BSL-3) laboratory conditions. The tests are quite expensive, and usually not done unless the symptoms are severe and remain so.

WHAT IS THE TREATMENT?

Treatment is aimed at minimizing the effects of symptoms. Acetaminophen (such as Tylenol) or paracetamol are used to treat fever and pain; lots of rest and liquids are also recommended. Health care workers in the area with cases should be contacted to be on the alert for more cases.

There is no vaccine for the disorder, although one is being tried in animal models. This disease is not one that can easily be controlled, even with a vaccine. The only way to prevent this disease is to prevent mosquito bites. The Centers for Disease Control and Prevention (CDC) recommends the following suggestions:

- Wear long-sleeved shirts, pants, and hats.
- Use insect repellent. Look for such ingredients as DEET, found in OFF!, Cutter, Sawyer, and Ultrathon. Picaridin is in Cutter Advances, Skin So Soft Bug Guard, and Skin Smart. Oil of lemon eucalyptus is an ingredient found in Repel and Off! Botanicals. IR3535 is in Skin So Soft Bug Guard Plus Expedition, and SkinSmart.
- Use permethrin-treated clothing and gear. Boots, pants, socks, and tents can be pre-treated. It is important to follow the manufacturer's directions.
- Stay and sleep in screened-in rooms.
- If one is outdoors, use mosquito netting and fans to keep mosquitoes away.
- Make sure that there is no standing water nearby. Mosquitoes breed in unsuspected places, even such an unsuspecting place as a cup of water.

For Further Information

Renn, Liam. *Chikungunya Virus—The New Reality: Your Next Vacation Could Make You Sick for Years.* Printed by Amazon Digital Services, 2015.

Creutzfeldt-Jakob Disease Variant: Human Mad Cow Disease

- Also known as variant Creutzfeldt-Jakob disease (vCJD), transmissible spongiform encephalopathy, bovine spongiform encephalopathy (in cattle)
- Deadly prion disease for which there is no treatment
- Since 1996, 229 cases of vCJD have been reported in 12 countries
- Transmitted by exposure to infected brain and nervous system tissues

In 1986 in Great Britain, cattle were dying. They were struck with a condition called bovine spongiform encephalopathy or mad cow disease, so named because of the behavior of the cattle. In 1996 the first case of a new human prion disease, called variant Creutzfeldt-Jakob (vCJD) disease, was diagnosed. A causal relationship was suspected between the cattle disease and the human condition. Many cattle were slaughtered. The first case in the United States was in December 2003.

The classic cases of CJD are spontaneous and may be hereditary; however vCJD is transmissible.

WHAT IS VARIANT CREUTZFELDT-JAKOB DISEASE?

vCJD is a disease of the brain and nervous system. It is transmitted by exposure to contaminated brain or nervous system tissue, possibly through the ingestion of meat with the abnormal prions or through certain medical procedures. Mad cow disease was discovered in the United Kingdom, and from 1986 to 2001, about 180,000 cattle were destroyed. The source of the cattle contamination was thought to be the production of bone meal, made from recycling dead and sick animals. Bone meal was then put into cattle feed. In 1996 in Great Britain, the first case of vCJD in humans was reported, and scientists believed the cause was eating contaminated meat.

The U.S. Department of Agriculture (USDA) confirmed a case of mad cow disease on a farm in Washington State in 2003, and the first person to die from vCJD in the United States occurred in June 2004. By May 2014, four people had died of vCJD in the United States. Worldwide, countries began to drastically change the feeding practices of cattle, and increased inspections. In March 2009, the United States banned the practice of using the brain and nervous systems material from cows who were too weak to stand (called downer cows) in cattle feed. As late as June 11, 2014, the USDA recalled 4,000 pounds of beef from a plant in Jackson, Missouri.

In order to understand vCJD, the symptoms and causes of classic CJD should also be presented. Actually, the two are the same disease, but transmitted differently. CJD belongs to a family of both human and animal diseases caused by prions. Prions are normal proteins in the brain that are not visible microscopically, contain no nucleic acid, and are highly resistant to destruction. However, if something changes these normal prion proteins, then an abnormal prion structure will develop. The abnormal form multiples and prevents the functioning of the normally structured proteins. This causes the death of brain cells. It produces a self-sustaining feedback loop as more and more prion proteins become abnormally structured. Dr. Stanley Prusiner of the University of California, San Francisco, won the Nobel Prize in physiology or medicine in 1997 for his discovery of prions.

The most common reason for this structural abnormality is a spontaneous change, but in some cases, genetic abnormalities may trigger the structural change. In the case of vCJD, the change is prompted by eating meat that contains these abnormally structured prions. Such procedures as corneal grafts, electrode implants, and immunoglobulin therapy have also been implicated in causing vCJD.

Prions also cause fatal familial insomnia (FFI) and Kuru, found among a tribe in Papua New Guinea, resulting from the ceremonial cannibalism practice of eating brains of the departed.

WHAT ARE THE SIGNS AND SYMPTOMS?

Regardless of how CJD is acquired, the symptoms are the same. It is a progressive, fatal disease. The first symptom is very rapid progressive dementia, in which the person has sudden loss of memory, personality changes, and hallucinations. The person may also be unusually agitated with mood swings, muscle stiffness, and involuntary jerky movements. Eventually, he or she may go blind, fall into a coma, and eventually die. The disease is always fatal. Most cases of classic CJD occur in people 60 and older, but vCJD is found in younger people and a longer period of time (perhaps as long as 50 years) occurs from the onset of symptoms to death.

HOW IS IT DIAGNOSED?

These symptoms are very similar to other progressive dementias, such as Alzheimer's disease or Huntington's disease. However, because of the changes in the brain tissue, deterioration is more rapid.

Like other dementias, there is no single diagnostic test or even combination of tests to conclusively prove the presence of vCJD. The physician must determine if the condition is actually one of the treatable forms of dementia. To do this, the following tools may be used: electroencephalogram (EEG) to measure brain electrical activity; brain magnetic resonance imaging (MRI); and lumbar puncture or spinal tap. vCJD can only be conclusively proved after an individual has died. A brain autopsy will reveal sponge-like holes throughout the brain

WHAT IS THE TREATMENT?

There is no treatment. The condition is always fatal. However, caregivers can give comfort and palliative care.

For Further Information

Prusiner, Stanley B. *Madness and Memory: The Discovery of Prions—A New Biological Principle of Disease.* New Haven, CT: Yale University Press, 2014.

Purdey, Mark. *Animal Pharm: One Man's Struggle to Discover the Truth about Mad Cow Disease and Variant CJD.* Sussex, UK: Clairview Books, 2008.

Cryptosporidiosis: Pain in the Stomach

- Caused by a protozoa
- Transmitted through contaminated drinking water or recreational water
- Can survive for long periods of time, even in chlorinated water
- One of the most common water-borne diseases

Seven-year-old Karen was very sick. She had watery diarrhea, nausea, and vomiting. Her parents thought she had stomach flu or had picked up something at school. But when the diarrhea did not go away into the third week, and some of her cousins also developed the condition, the doctor looked for an explanation. All the children had swum in the same pool a few weeks before. When her stools were analyzed, they showed a parasite called *Cryptosporidium*. Karen had picked up the parasite from the contaminated water in the pool.

Although this one-celled organism is found in hot tubs, fountains, lakes, rivers, ponds, and streams, as well as in swimming pools, it is one that people are generally not aware of.

WHAT IS CRYPTOSPORIDIOSIS?

The parasite *Cryptosporidium* is a protozoa that is found in the fecal matter of infected people or animals. If an infected person or animal defecates in the water, the parasite thrives in the water and can infect other people. The protozoa have very tough oocysts or shells that allow them to survive in the environment. It can even survive for days in properly chlorinated pools.

This tiny microscopic organism was not identified until 1976, but is one of the most common parasites found worldwide. It is especially a problem for three groups of people: young children, pregnant women, and people with compromised immune systems.

Infection can occur in several ways, but all are traced back to the contaminated water. It is not spread through the air or blood but must be transferred to the mouth and swallowed. People can pick up crypto from many sources. The main one appears to be swallowing contaminated recreational water, such as in a pool. One can get the disorder by putting anything in the mouth, such as food that has come in contact with feces of an infected person. In addition, one can pick up crypto from lounge chairs, picnic tables, bathroom fixtures, and changing tables that have been touched by an individual with crypto. In 1987, 13,000 people in Carrollton, Georgia became ill with crypto, spread through the municipal water system that met all federal drinking water standards.

WHAT ARE THE SIGNS AND SYMPTOMS?

One of the key symptoms is watery diarrhea. The symptoms appear between two and ten days after exposure, with an average onset of seven days. In addition, the person may have stomach cramps, vomiting, nausea, and a low fever. Children, pregnant women, and those who are immunocompromised can develop a more severe form of crypto.

The organism takes up residence in the intestinal wall and can stay there for an extended period of time. Even people with no symptoms can pass the parasite on. For those with seriously compromised immune systems, such as those with AIDS, the parasite may spread beyond the intestines and infiltrate the lungs, middle ear, pancreas, liver, and stomach. When this occurs, it can be fatal.

HOW IS IT DIAGNOSED?

When the condition is suspected, several tests can identify the organism. The technician should examine at least three stool samples, using special staining techniques that reveal oocysts under the microscope. A second method is to detect antibodies using blood analysis. A third procedure uses polymerase chain reaction (PCR), which can identify the specific species of *Cryptosporidium*. The latter tests are usually performed on people who have some immune-compromising disorder such as AIDS.

CRYPTO: THE MOST COMMON WATER-BORNE INFECTION

Crypto, the most common water-borne infection, can be prevented and avoided with certain actions. Remember that the organism can stay alive for days, even in well-maintained pools. Knowledge about the cause and prevention is important. According to the Centers for Disease Control and Prevention (CDC), one must take the following actions:

- All swimmers should be aware of the potential for crypto, and never swallow or drink the water that they swim in.
- Keep feces and urine out of the water.
- Do not swim if you have diarrhea.
- Shower with soap before you start swimming and rinse or shower any time you leave the water and get back in.
- Wash your hands after going to the bathroom.
- Before getting in the pool, check that the chlorine level is at 1–3 mg/L or ppm, and pH should be 7.2–7.8. You can purchase these measuring devices at superstores or pool supply stores.
- For parents of young children, take them to the bathroom every 30-60 minutes; change diapers in an area designated for changing and not at poolside.

WHAT IS THE TREATMENT?

For those with a healthy immune system, crypto will usually resolve on its own. Individuals should stay well-hydrated to mitigate the effects of prolonged diarrhea. For those with compromised immune systems, certain antibiotics and other medications may be given, but these treatments do not always work. A vaccine that has been tested on a mouse model is being developed, because the spores do produce an antigen.

For Further Information

Chen, X. M., J. S. Keithly, C. V. Paya, and N. F. LaRusso. 2002. "Current Concepts: Cryptosporidiosis." *New England Journal of Medicine* 346 (22): 1723–31.

Cutaneous Larva Migrans (CLM): When the Skin Creeps

- Also known as creeping eruption; ground itch; sand worm; plumber's itch
- Skin disease caused by the larvae of the dog and cat hookworm
- Causes severe itching and burning
- Will appear as if something is creeping in different directions under the skin

A child plays in her backyard sandbox. Her unsuspecting parents do not know that the neighborhood cats visited the uncovered sand box sometime during the night. After several hours, the child begins to cry. Her feet are burning and itching and her mother notes a red area around the toes. The child wants to scratch; some topical ointment may help the pain. But soon, mom notices that there are raised streaks that begin to run across the areas of the toes and up onto the foot. This child has a condition called cutaneous larva migrans.

WHAT IS CUTANEOUS LARVA MIGRANS?

Cutaneous larva migrans (CLM) is a skin disease caused by the larvae of the dog and cat hookworm. The hookworm eggs are passed in feces and hatch into larvae in the warm soil. The larvae burrow into exposed skin, and because they cannot get into a human's circulatory system, they stay just under the top layers of the skin, causing an itchy mass that runs in streaks as the larvae migrate under the skin.

Hookworms are parasites that live in the intestines of the host. They are members of the family of roundworms or nematodes called *Ancyclostomatidae*. The adult worms have special structures that hook onto the intestinal walls of the host and get their nourishment from the bloodstream. There they lay eggs, which are excreted in the feces of the animal. In the soil, especially warm sand, the eggs hatch out into a larval or filariform stage. These larvae live in the soil until they come in contact with some type of flesh.

Sandy beaches are optimal places for larval development. And it is not just children who may get the infection. Any person who walks along an area without shoes or who sits on the ground may pick up the larvae. Plumbers, electricians, contractors, farmers, or anyone who works in the soil has the potential to get this infection.

The larvae can only burrow through the outer layer of the skin (the epidermis) and into the top layer of the dermis. There it is stopped, because this species of hookworm does not have the enzymes that can break through to the deeper levels and allow the larvae into the bloodstream. Thus, the larvae grow and multiply just under the skin, burrowing in many directions under the skin.

The condition is common in tropical and subtropical climates; however, it can occur in temperate climates in warmer months. The highest incidence in the United States is in Florida. Travelers should know that CLM is indigenous to the Caribbean, Central and South America, Southeast Asia, and Australia.

WHAT ARE THE SIGNS AND SYMPTOMS?

The red area swells, itches, and burns like it is on fire. Scratching with the fingernails may cause a secondary bacterial infection. The pathways of the larvae under the skin are very visible. They appear like little snakes running in different directions under the skin.

HOW IS IT DIAGNOSED?

The person with the parasite will notice that something is burning and itching on the skin. There is a red eruption that appears to be running in different directions. The person will go to the doctor for treatment because of the itchiness, and a doctor can usually pinpoint the cause simply through physical examination due to the condition's distinctive symptoms.

WHAT IS THE TREATMENT?

Doctors treat CLM in several ways:

- Medications may be given by mouth; these prescriptions will then be excreted through the skin, killing the larvae. These agents include albendazole (Albenza) and ivermectin (Stromectol)
- Thiabendazole (Mintezol) can be taken orally or topically by grinding the pills and applying with petroleum jelly. The oral preparations may have serious side effects, and the topical treatment may be preferred.

- Application of an anti-itch cream such as cortisone or calamine lotion may relieve the itch.
- An antibiotic cream may be recommended for secondary infections caused by scratching.

Wearing shoes is recommended to prevent infections. In some areas, beaches may ban dogs during certain seasons. It is essential that all pets be checked for worms, take preventive medications that are available, and be treated if they are infected.

For Further Information
Caumes, E. 2000. "Treatment of Cutaneous Larva Migrans." *Clinical Infectious Diseases* 30 (5): 811–814.

Dengue Fever: A Disease That Feels Like "Breaking Bones"

- Also known as break bone fever; break heart fever; La dengue; dengue hemorrhagic fever; dengue shock syndrome; bilious remitting fever
- A mosquito-borne viral infection
- Can cause mild symptoms or a more severe reaction, including massive internal hemorrhaging
- Once thought eradicated in the United States, but now reemerging

Marjory Stoneman Douglas in *Everglades: River of Grass* describes life in Miami, Florida in 1915 when it was a little community of 5,000 people. She refers to epidemics of dengue, or break bone fever. Florida, as well as many places in the South, had severe outbreaks of dengue fever. The cities were stricken by the fever with major epidemics in the following years: Charleston, South Carolina, 1828; Savannah, Georgia, 1850; Austin, Texas, 1885; Galveston, Texas, 1897; most of Louisiana, 1922; and Miami, Florida, 1934. Once the federal government undertook mass mosquito eradication and education programs, dengue fever was all but eliminated. The last serious outbreak in the United States was in Miami in 1934.

Recently, the Centers for Disease Control and Prevention (CDC) has expressed concern over new outbreaks of dengue. In July 2009, a case was confirmed in Miami, Florida. The woman had not traveled out of the area. In 2013 dengue was detected in Martin County, Florida, a coastal area about 100 miles north of Miami. About 18 cases have appeared in this county, and in another county to the north.

WHAT IS DENGUE FEVER?

Dengue is a viral infection carried by mosquitoes, and until recently was found only in tropical and subtropical regions. The mosquito carries four different but closely related types of the virus: DEN-1, DEN-2, DEN-3, and DEN-4. Dengue can be either mild or severe. Severe dengue is also known as dengue hemorrhagic fever and dengue shock fever.

Several species of *Aedes* mosquito cause the disease, but *Aedes aegypti* and *Aedes albopictus* are the most common. *Aedes aegypti* thrives in urban areas and breeds in humanmade containers where water has collected. The female mosquito lays her eggs in standing water—even a small cup can provide a breeding ground. Old tires collecting water are infamous breeding areas. The mosquito can bite many different people in one feeding period. *Aedes albopictus* has spread from Asia through international trade and travel and is adaptable to more temperate climates.

The virus lives in the cells that line the mosquito's intestine, but then in about 10 days, migrates to the saliva. The mosquito then injects the virus into another person when it bites. Humans are the prime target, but dengue can also be found in certain nonhuman primates. The mosquito is infected for life.

Dengue fever is endemic in more than 110 countries and is now considered a global problem. Each year, over 100 million cases occur is such areas as India, Southeast Asia, Southeast China and Taiwan, islands in the Pacific, the Caribbean (except Cuba and the Caiman Islands), Mexico, Africa, and Central and South America. Dengue was endemic in the southern part of the United States until about 1935. However, there appears to be a resurgence in the United States.

A Chinese medical book from the Jin Dynasty about 265–420 AD is perhaps the earliest written account of dengue. The slave trade that began in the 16th century brought dengue to the New World. Many epidemics were reported in the United States, with serious outbreaks in 1779 and 1780. In 1906, the *Aedes* mosquito was identified as the carrier, and in 1907, dengue was shown to be caused by a virus. John Burton Cleland (1878–1971), an Australian pathologist, and Franklin Siler (1875–1960) described how the disease was transmitted. Siler was an army physician who was noted for investigating dengue fever in the Philippines.

Dengue is a Spanish word that possibly came from a Swahili word *dinga*, meaning "caused by an evil spirit."

WHAT ARE THE SIGNS AND SYMPTOMS?

Dengue fever is divided into two classes: dengue fever and severe dengue fever. It may begin with a high fever, but then several additional symptoms may be present: severe headache with pain behind the eyes, vomiting, nausea, swollen glands, rash, mild bleeding from nose or gums, low white blood cell count, or severe joint or muscle pain may appear. It is the muscle and joint pain that gives it the nickname "break bone fever."

Symptoms usually appear within four to 10 days after a bite from an infected mosquito, and usually last from seven to 10 days. The condition is different from many other diseases in that young children and those with their first infection have milder symptoms than older children and adults.

Severe dengue can occur if the fever does not go down in three to seven days. Warning signs of serious complications include the following:

- Severe pain in the abdomen with persistent vomiting, especially of blood
- Red rash on the skin
- Profuse bleeding from the nose or gums
- Irritability and drowsiness
- Pale, cold, clammy skin
- Difficulty breathing

These signs indicate that the person has developed dengue hemorrhagic fever (DHF) and has internal bleeding and leakage of blood plasma into the abdominal cavity or into the cavities surrounding the lungs. This loss of fluid may lead to failure of the circulatory system and death. Another serious condition is dengue shock syndrome, in which fluid loss causes blood pressure to drop dangerously low. At one time these two were considered separate disorders, but now are classified together as severe dengue.

Milder dengue fever has a mortality rate of less than 1 percent, and even severe dengue fever has a mortality rate of only about 5 percent if proper supportive medical care is given. However, without any medical treatment, the mortality rate of DHF can be as high as 50 percent.

HOW IS IT DIAGNOSED?

Those with milder forms of dengue may not seek medical attention. However, if a physician is consulted, he or she will likely ask the patient about their recent health history, including any travel to areas where dengue is endemic. A blood test can confirm if the person is afflicted with dengue.

WHAT IS THE TREATMENT?

There is no cure and no vaccine. Milder symptoms can be minimized with pain relievers, fluids, and rest. Medical treatment for severe cases focuses on preventing organ failure and death. Researchers are working on both a medical cure and a vaccine, but currently these are in trials. The best treatment is prevention.

PREVENTING DENGUE AND OTHER
MOSQUITO-BORNE INFECTIONS

People are traveling more these days. Cruises to the Caribbean and Central America are especially popular. However, one needs to be aware that any tropical or subtropical region can have mosquitoes that are possibly infected with dengue. The Centers for Disease Control and Prevention (CDC) makes the following suggestions:

- Cover your skin with clothing. Shoes, socks, long pants, and long sleeves are suggested.
- Use mosquito repellent. Apply both to bare skin and clothing. Repellents include DEET, picaridin, and oil of lemon eucalyptus.
- Around your home, remove mosquito breeding places by draining any standing water.
- Make sure swimming pools are properly maintained and chlorinated; empty plastic swimming pools when not in use.
- Make sure all screens are in good repair.
- Use mosquito repellent candles and coils for outside events.

For Further Information

Gubler, Duane J., Eng Eong Ooi, and Subhash Vasudevan, eds. *Dengue and Dengue Hemorrhagic Fever*. Oxfordshire, UK: CABI, 2014.

Ebola: Bleeding from All Body Openings

- Also known as Ebola virus disease (EVD); Ebola hemorrhagic fever (EHF)
- Outbreaks mainly in sub-Saharan Africa; most recently in 2014
- Mortality as high as 90 percent
- Causes internal and external bleeding through all body openings

Much attention has focused recently on Ebola in developing countries of Africa. The largest, most recent, and still ongoing outbreak of this deadly disease began in 2014, and has since spread to six African countries, including Liberia, Mali, and Senegal. A few cases were also reported in nations such as the United States, United Kingdom, and Spain, when missionaries and health care workers returned home for treatment. In total, almost 26,000 people have been infected, and almost 11,000 have died.

WHAT IS EBOLA?

Ebola virus disease is a highly lethal condition caused by any of five Ebola viruses.

Ebola is known as a hemorrhagic virus. Ebola causes the blood vessels in the internal organs to break and bleed, and blood flows out of all body orifices and openings, including the mouth, nose, rectum, and urinary tract. Of the five known strains of Ebola, all of them have similar hemorrhagic properties.

The virus belongs to a group of viruses called filoviruses. The Ebola virus consists of only one molecule of single-stranded RNA enclosed in a lipid envelope. Like other viruses, Ebola invades and takes over the host's cells. The invaded cells produce a protein called Ebola virus protein, which attaches to the inside of blood vessels. This attachment then causes the lining of the vessels to break, causing hemorrhaging. The viral protein also keeps the blood from clotting adding to the internal bleeding. When the immune system tries to react, the neutrophils, a type of white blood cell, are blocked. In fact, the virus may connect to the neutrophil and travel with it to other parts of the body, such as the brain, liver, and other organs.

At present, Ebola is contained within the continent of Africa. Although outbreaks could have occurred in the past, the first identified outbreak happened in Yambuku in the northern Congo in 1976. The name "Ebola" comes from the Ebola River, in the north of the Republic of the Congo. At the same time, an outbreak occurred in Zaire. This Zaire strain killed 90 percent of the people who contracted it.

Baron Dr. Peter Piot (1949–) from the Netherlands is Professor of Health at the London School of Hygiene and Tropical Medicine. Dr. Piot was a member of the team who was sent to Zaire in 1976, when he discovered the virus. His efforts are described in his book *No Time to Lose: A Life in Pursuit of Deadly Viruses,* in which he laments that even after many outbreaks, we still know too little about the virus and how to treat it.

Scientists have worked tirelessly to locate the source of the Ebola virus. Traces of the virus have been found in chimpanzees and gorillas, but because these animals die from hemorrhagic bleeding, they are probably not the host. The most likely vector agent is the fruit bat. These flying animals are known to harbor many viruses, and because they move from area to area, they can spread the disease quickly. The flying bats drop bits of fruit on the ground, and animals such as gorillas and rats feed on these fruits. Scientists think that the saliva of the bat carries the virus. Humans in many of the areas of the world eat bush meat such as bats, rats, and monkeys and thus may contract the virus. During the recent outbreaks, several governments banned eating bush meat.

The virus is easily transmitted from human to human through body fluids, especially if one touches the mouth or eyes. The virus does not appear to be spread by droplets or aerosols in the air. Injections from unsterilized needles and contact with bodily fluids are also a means of transmission. Touching the bodies of the dead, a funeral practice in some areas of Africa, also helps spread the virus.

Ironically, the speed with which Ebola is transmitted and its quick and high mortality actually help contain outbreaks and prevent them from spreading farther.

WHAT ARE THE SIGNS AND SYMPTOMS?

Ebola strikes suddenly. The person may think he or she has a bad case of influenza with a quick onset of fever, chills, aching in joints and muscles, and chest pain. The person is nauseated and then develops pain in the abdomen, along with diarrhea and vomiting. The respiratory system is now involved—a very sore throat, cough, and difficulty breathing develop. The person is confused, apathetic, and may have seizures or fall into a coma. The skin may have a rash and develop large hematomas around needle injection sites. Blood will begin to seep from all orifices. The internal bleeding is especially noted from the gastrointestinal tract.

Mortality rates vary based on the particular strain of Ebola. Some are as low as 25 percent, while the Zaire strain is as high as 90 percent. The overall risk of death is approximately 50 percent. Death, when it occurs, usually happens six to 16 days after symptoms first appear. Recovery is usually quick and complete and may impart immunity from subsequent reinfection.

HOW IS IT DIAGNOSED?

The first symptoms of Ebola are very much like those of other conditions, and so either medical care may not be sought (if it is even available), or a doctor may misdiagnose the condition. Ebola may be suspected if there is a current outbreak. Although the virus can be detected in the blood, diagnosis is usually done only to confirm suspicions once telltale symptoms such as hemorrhaging have begun. And, because it may take some time to determine if Ebola is present in the blood and the virus can kill so quickly, such diagnostic tools are not always practical. Additionally, doctors in areas where Ebola may occur may not be equipped with the necessary diagnostic tests.

WHAT IS THE TREATMENT?

The U.S. Food and Drug Administration (FDA) has not approved any therapy for Ebola. Treatment is supportive and may include pain management, hydration, and blood transfusions. Current cures and vaccines are under investigation.

For Further Information
Preston, Richard. *The Hot Zone*. New York: Anchor Books, 2014.

Elephantiasis: Swollen Arms and Legs

- Also known as lymphatic filariasis; Barbados leg; elephant leg; morbis herculeus
- Affects over 120 million people in 73 countries
- Caused by specific nematodes or roundworms known as filarial worms
- Causes massive swelling in arms and legs

It only takes one picture of a person with the enormous swelling of the legs and feet to remember elephantiasis. The limbs or body parts swell so much that they resemble an elephant's foreleg in size, texture, and color. Although the disease is not currently seen in the United States, it is an important problem in many parts of the world.

WHAT IS ELEPHANTIASIS?

Also known as lymphatic filariasis, this disease is the result of a parasitic infection by the filarial worm. These worms, also called nematodes or round worms, have a long thread-like shape and are found mostly in tropical and subtropical regions. Eight filarial worms are known to affect humans, and they are classified in three groups: cutaneous, lymphatic, and abdominal cavity worms. The lymphatic filaria cause elephantiasis. The most common lymphatic filarial are *Wuchereria bancrofti* (in about 90 percent of cases) and *Brugia malayi*.

Several kinds of mosquitoes carry different forms of the roundworm, but the effect of each one is similar. Examples of the mosquitoes that carry these worms are *Aedes aegypti,* which carries malaria and other disorders, *Anopheles,* and *Culex.*

The worm is transmitted from person to person. A mosquito bites an infected person and picks up the larvae of the adult worm from the body of the person; these are called microfilaria, and these tiny forms infect the mosquito. Then the infected female mosquito injects the larvae into another individual while biting, and these small worms migrate up a lymphatic channel. During this time they develop and become adult worms. The development can take from a few months to years, as the worms grow to about one to four inches long. The adult worms have been known to live from three to eight years. Adult worms constantly produce the tiny microfilaria, which can be picked up by other mosquitoes and passed on to others.

The lymphatic system is the network of vessels through which lymph drains from the tissues into the blood. The symptoms of elephantiasis are caused when the lymphatic system is blocked by the worms.

The condition affects over 120 million people in 73 countries in regions including Asia, Africa, the Western Pacific, parts of the Caribbean, and South America.

The last known case in the United States was in Charleston, South Carolina, in the early 20th century.

WHAT ARE THE SIGNS AND SYMPTOMS?

Although most people that have the condition never develop the clinical symptoms, for the small percentage that do develop symptoms, it becomes quite noticeable. Upon infection, the body reacts with fever, shaking, chills, sweating, vomiting, and pain. After that, the lymph nodes enlarge with swelling of the affected areas and development of skin ulcers. Abscesses at the area of the lymph nodes may develop in the hard and thickened skin. Most commonly, the swelling begins in the ankle and then progresses to the leg and foot. Elephantiasis causes enormous swelling in the arms, legs, and the genitals. The skin may appear dark with warty-like growths; if these areas crack, infection can set in. The disorder is very disabling and disfiguring.

HOW IS IT DIAGNOSED?

Elephantiasis can easily be suspected if a patient presents with the telltale swelling. However, the only sure way to diagnose the condition is to detect the parasite in the person's blood, which can be done only in certain ways. The blood must be collected during the night when the microfilaria are the most numerous and are migrating. The adult worms are usually difficult to detect because they are deep in the lymphatic system.

WHAT IS THE TREATMENT?

The person must be given a strong drug that kills both the microfilaria and the adult worms. The drug diethylcarbamazine (DEC) or Hetrazan is taken in tablet form. However, the body reacts to the dead and dying worms, so the person must be carefully monitored. Another drug, Ivermectin, is being studied, but may not kill the adult worm as effectively. Surgery may be performed to drain lymph from the swollen areas and remove dead worms.

To prevent the disease, individuals should avoid being bitten by mosquitoes. This includes wearing protective clothing and using insect repellent, as well as removing possible breeding areas for mosquitoes. Most of the people with elephantiasis are bitten by many mosquitoes. It is rare for tourists visiting the infected areas for only a short time to pick up these worms.

For Further Information

Hoerauf, Achim, et al. 2003. "Doxycycline as a Novel Strategy against Bancroftian Filariasis—Depletion of Qolbachia Endosymbionts from Wuchereria Bancrofti and Stop of Microfilaria Production." *Medical Microbiology and Immunology* 192 (4): 211–6.

Enterovirus-D68: Outbreak of a Rare Virus

- Also known as EV-D68; Human enterovirus 68
- First identified in California in 1962; since then only about 100 cases noted until 2014
- Symptoms start like a common cold, then progress rapidly into a respiratory infection
- No specific treatments available

In the fall of 2014, a virus called human enterovirus 68 startled health officials. One father described the condition by saying that his son went from a having a cold to being probably minutes away from death. The father was describing his teenage son's bout with EV-D68.

This virus caused hundreds of children to be hospitalized in nine states from California to Georgia. What is so unusual about this, is that since its discovery in 1962, there have been only 100 cases traced to this virus. In Kansas City alone, more than 450 children went to Children's Mercy Hospital, and 60 of them received intensive care at the hospital. At the Colorado Children's Hospital, more than 900 children were seen in a two week period in August 2014. What is this virus that has suddenly emerged? It is called human enterovirus D68 or EV-D68.

WHAT IS ENTEROVIRUS-D68?

Enterovirus-D68 (EV-D68) is called a nonpolio enterovirus. In the 1950s, the virus that causes poliomyelitis (polio) shattered the lives of children and some adults and left them physically handicapped. This virus is one of more than 100 nonpolio enteroviruses that appear to have mutated to cause serious lung and respiratory infections. Previously, only a few cases had been reported since its identification in 1962.

People are more likely to get this virus in summer and fall. This virus is like other viruses; it is spread by person-to-person contact. Because it is found in saliva, nasal mucus, and sputum, it is spread when the person sneezes or coughs, as particles are projected through the air. The virus also lives for a short period of time on objects and surfaces, so if a person touches these, he or she may pick up the virus.

The people most at risk are infants, children, and teenagers. Adults may get the infection, but it is less likely to cause a severe illness.

WHAT ARE THE SIGNS AND SYMPTOMS?

EV-D68 symptoms range from mild to severe respiratory illness. The symptoms start out like a cold. The child may be sneezing, have a runny nose, and a cough. Some of the children with the virus get over it with just cold-like symptoms. But then others develop a severe cough, have difficulty breathing, and/or develop a rash. This is when one should immediately go to the doctor. Children that have asthma or a compromised immune system are especially susceptible for a severe case.

HOW IS IT DIAGNOSED?

Swabs of the person's nose or throat can specifically determine EV-D68. On October 14, 2014, the Centers for Disease Control and Prevention (CDC) developed a new, faster test for detecting the virus. This now can be done within a few days.

WHAT IS THE TREATMENT?

There are no specific treatments for enteroviruses. The main thing is to control the symptoms to make the person more comfortable. The standard of plenty of rest, fluids, and over-the counter medications are recommended. However, those with severe cases that are admitted to the hospital will receive assistance in breathing and other therapies to help build up the immune system.

The best treatment is like that of other communicable diseases: prevention by taking a few common sense precautions. Handwashing for 20 seconds is very important, especially after going to the bathroom. Clean and disinfect objects that are touched often by people. And avoid shaking hands, hugging, or sharing items with those who are sick. Individuals should also stay home from work or school if they are ill.

For Further Information

Clark, James. *Enterovirus: The Preppers Guide to Surviving Enterovirus*. Printed by Amazon Digital Services, 2014.

Hantavirus: Mystery Disease Carried by Mice

- Formerly known as Four Corners disease and Sin Nombre virus
- RNA virus carried by rodents
- Two types: pulmonary and hemorrhagic
- Mortality rate as high as 38 percent

Four Corners is an area of the United States shared by the states of Arizona, New Mexico, Colorado, and Utah. Much of the area contains the Navajo Native American Reservation. In 1993, a young, healthy Navajo man was rushed to a hospital in New Mexico breathing very hard; he soon died. The medical personnel remembered that a few days before, a young woman with similar symptoms had died. This woman happened to be the man's fiancée. Investigators soon found that in the same area, five other healthy young people had died, all of whom had the same symptoms. When additional cases came in, they realized that they were dealing with a mystery virus. That virus was found to be hantavirus.

WHAT IS HANTAVIRUS?

Hantavirus is a member of the virus family called *Bunyaviridae*. The viruses infect rats and mice, but these animals do not get the disease. There are two basic types of hantavirus: one causes hemorrhagic disease with kidney failure syndrome (HFRS); this virus is found primarily in Asia, Europe, and Africa. The second type is hantavirus pulmonary syndrome (HPS), affecting the lungs. This type is found in North, Central, and South America. Human infections are related to contact with rodents.

The hantavirus is a relative newcomer to the genus of viruses. The name hantavirus comes from an area around the Hantan River in South Korea. During the Korean War (1950–1953), American and Korean soldiers became ill with generalized hemorrhage or bleeding, shock, and renal failure. In 1976, virologists Ho-Wang Lee and Karl M. Johnson began the search that ended in the isolation of the virus in striped field mice. In 1993, the outbreak at Four Corners was from the strain of virus that infects the lungs. Weeks later the virus known as Sin Nombre, which is Spanish for "nameless," was found to be carried by a rodent host, the deer mouse.

Rodents carry all strains of hantavirus. The virus is found in urine and feces. Humans get sick when they come in contact with rodent urine or feces. For example, one may be cleaning homes, sheds, or other areas that have been empty for a long time. Outdoor hikers and campers who spend the night in a wooded area may come in contact with droppings on the ground. The particles become aerosolized on the dust and breathed in by humans. Most researchers agree that it does not spread between humans, though one type in Argentina is suspected to be transmitted by person-to-person contact.

The virus has three single-stranded RNA segments. Each virion (one of the viruses) is very small and can be easily aerosolized.

The question of why there was a sudden escalation of cases in the Four Corners region was answered in the study of the population of deer mice. The Four Corners area had been in a drought for many years, but in 1993, heavy snows melted and helped drought-stricken plants and animals to thrive. The deer mice population exploded, helping to spread the virus among the rodents, then to humans.

The most recent outbreak was at Curry Village in Yosemite National Park in 2012. Hantavirus infected at least 10 people and killed three. Warnings were put out through other national park camps.

WHAT ARE THE SIGNS AND SYMPTOMS?

Although both types of hantavirus are carried by rodents, they present with different symptoms. In the case of HFRS, individuals present with fever, bleeding from orifices, and kidney failure. More than 3,000 soldiers became ill from this condition during the Korean War, and 10 percent died. The pulmonary type that is the one found at Four Corners has since been found throughout the United States. The symptoms start out very much like the flu with chills, fever, headache, and muscle aches. In one or two days, the person finds breathing is becoming very difficult. He or she has a dry cough, headache, nausea, vomiting, and a general feeling of illness. It differs from other lung infections like influenza or pneumonia in that fluid that builds up is clear and does not have yellow or pus-like inflammation. Death occurs in about 38 percent of patients, either as the result of lung failure for the pulmonary type or kidney failure for the hemorrhagic type.

HOW IS IT DIAGNOSED?

A physical exam will reveal lung or kidney issues, low blood pressure, or low oxygen levels that may cause the skin to turn blue. The health care provider will ask about the person's association with rodents or potential contact with airborne contamination. Tests include blood tests to check for hantavirus, a complete blood count (CBC), complete metabolic panel, kidney and liver function tests, X-ray of chest, and a CT scan of chest.

WHAT IS THE TREATMENT?

If it has been determined that a person has hantavirus, he or she is admitted to the hospital and possibly put in intensive care. Here he or she will be given oxygen, a medication called ribavirin if there are kidney-related problems, and special machines to oxygenate the blood. All of the treatment is intended to avoid the complications of kidney or heart and lung failure.

Research is being done to develop a safe and effective hantavirus vaccine. One problem in developing this is that there is no animal model for study. Models usually include mice, but the virus does not produce symptoms in rodents. The Korean Army does use a vaccine, but the U.S. Food and Drug Administration (FDA) and World Health Organization (WHO) have not approved a vaccine for hantavirus.

PREVENTING HANTAVIRUS

The National Park Service and the National Institutes of Health offer these suggestions for prevention.

1. When hiking and camping, pitch tents in areas where there are no rodent droppings; rodents will bed in woodpiles and dense brush.
2. Take care not to stir up dust.
3. Sleep on a ground cover and pad and not directly on the ground; try to sleep at least 12 inches off the ground or in a tent with flooring.
4. Avoid touching live or dead rodents, and avoid their burrows and nests.
5. Keep food in tightly sealed containers and store away from rodents.
6. Dispose of all trash promptly in accordance with park rules, or pack in rodent-proof containers.

Since most of the infections come from homes, the following applies to these:

1. Keep your home clean. Clear out potential nesting sites, especially in the kitchen
2. When opening an unused cabin, shed, or other building, open all doors and windows, leave the building, and allow for the space to air out about 30 minutes.
3. When you return to the building, spray the surfaces with a disinfectant.
4. Spray mouse nests with 10 percent solution of chlorine bleach. Using rubber gloves, place the materials in plastic bags and dispose of all materials.

For Further Information

Johnson, K. M. 2001. "Hantaviruses: history and overview." *Current Topics in Microbiology and Immunology* 256: 1–14.

Herpes Zoster: From Chickenpox to Shingles

- Causes both chickenpox and shingles
- Chickenpox is a very communicable, airborne virus, once common during childhood
- Latent virus lives in the nerves and may be activated under certain conditions as shingles
- Shingles is very painful; ranges from 1.2 to 3.2 cases per 1,000 healthy individuals

Sharon has had back surgeries, cardiac surgery, and breast cancer, and has dealt often with pain. However, when she developed a rash that traveled around her waist to her back, she commented that of all the conditions that she had never had, nothing was as painful as shingles. She thought it was unusual when the doctor asked if she had chickenpox as a child. She found out that the disease that was causing so much pain was caused by the herpes zoster virus, which she had had as a six-year-old in the form of chickenpox. It was still present in her system, and causing the disorder called shingles.

WHAT IS HERPES ZOSTER?

Herpes zoster, known also as varicella zoster virus (VZV), is a double-stranded piece of DNA, and a member of the same genus as *Herpes simplex,* the virus that causes cold sores and fever blisters. *Herpes zoster* causes chickenpox, a disease once common during childhood. It is a well-known airborne, communicable disease that schoolchildren pass around. When the chickenpox symptoms disappear, the child's immune system has eliminated most of the viruses except for just a few that have migrated along nerves to settle in the dorsal root ganglion, a network of nerve cells near the spinal cord. Called latent viruses, they remain in the nerve network forever, and may be activated later in life, at which point the condition is known as shingles. Why this happens sometimes but not always is still unknown.

Chickenpox has been around for a long time. The first recorded instance was in 1684. The origin of the term "chickenpox" is debatable. Some people think that it arose because the lesions looked like chickpeas; others said that the lesions resembled the pecks that might be made by the chicken pecking in the dirt. Others proposed that it is a corruption of the term "itching-pox."

Shingles or zona caused by *Herpes zoster* also has a long recorded history although most accounts believe that people confused the disorder with smallpox, ergotism (caused by eating food contaminated with a fungus), or erysipelas (red rash patches caused by a bacteria). In the eighteenth century, William Heberden (1710–1801) determined the difference between herpes zoster and smallpox; in the late 19th century, it was shown to be different from erysipelas. In the 19th century, Richard Bright (1789–1858) and Felix von Bärensprung (1822–1864) discovered that it arose from the dorsal root ganglion. However, the realization that the two were caused by the same virus did not gain strength until Nobel Laureate Thomas Huckle Weller (1915–2008) isolated the varicella virus in cell cultures in 1953.

The name "shingles" comes from Latin word *cingulum*, meaning belt or girdle that goes round the waist. Shingles often erupts around the waist area.

The risk factors for shingles include the following:

- The person is over 60 and had chickenpox as a child.
- A special risk factor occurs if the person had chickenpox before the age of one year.

- The person has a weakened immune system from some other condition such as AIDS or medications.

Some people have pain in the area even after all symptoms have disappeared. This is called post-herpetic pain.

WHAT ARE THE SIGNS AND SYMPTOMS?

Chickenpox. For young children, usually there are no early symptoms (called pro-dromal symptoms). The child acts irritable and fussy, but generally not enough for the parent to think that the child has a communicable disease. The rash then breaks out. It begins as small dots on the face, hands, torso, or back, and then progresses to lesion-like blisters within about 10 to 12 hours. The lesions scab over and eventually fall off. The most irritating problem is that the blisters may itch, and the child wants to scratch. Because there are so few warnings, one can see how this communicable disease can spread rapidly through schools and other places.

For adolescents and adults, chickenpox has distinct prodromal symptoms. The person may lose appetite, become nauseous, and have aching muscles, along with a splitting headache. He or she may think that it's the flu. Then the blisters break out. In addition to the body trunk, the blisters may be on the palms, soles of feet, and genital area. Sores in the mouth and throat can be painful and itchy and make it difficult to swallow. The rash can be both internal and external and is widespread; the fever lasts longer than in children. In addition, adults may have more complications, such as varicella pneumonia.

If a person never had chickenpox as a child and is exposed to the virus, he or she will likely develop chickenpox. When a pregnant woman contracts chickenpox, it is especially dangerous, because the varicella virus can seriously affect the fetus and cause brain, eye, or skin disorders.

Shingles. The first symptoms usually include a headache or sensitivity to light. The person thinks that he or she has the flu, but there is no fever. Then small red patches that are painful appear usually on one side of the body. The patches develop fluid-filled blisters that break easily and crust over. It takes about two to four weeks for the blisters to heal. If the rash is on the face, it can also invade the eyes and cause serious vision problems. If the shingles infection is on the face or near the eyes, a condition called Ramsay Hunt syndrome can occur in which damage to the facial nerve leads to facial paralysis and hearing loss.

HOW IS IT DIAGNOSED?

A physician can diagnose most cases by simple physical examination. There are additional tests that can be done in certain circumstances, but these are rare.

WHAT IS THE TREATMENT?

For childhood chickenpox, relieving the itching is probably the most important thing. The child's fingernails should be cut short. Gloves may be used to combat scratching. Over-the-counter treatment with calamine lotion or cold compresses can reduce itching.

Shingles has no cure, but it can be treated to ease pain and shorten symptoms. The person should go to a health care provider as soon as the symptoms of shingles appear. Treatment for shingles involves taking antiviral medicines such as acyclovir. Anti-inflammation drugs and narcotic medications also may reduce pain and swelling. Certain numbing creams, gels, or patches can relieve pain. If pain continues after the patches have cleared, zostrix cream can relieve this pain. Proper home care is essential. The person must get a lot of rest, apply cold compresses to the rash, and take colloidal oatmeal baths to relieve pain.

Today, there is a vaccine for both chickenpox and shingles, both of which have been available since 1995. Although chickenpox was once a common childhood illness, the extensive use of the vaccine have all but eliminated it as a disease among American children. For adults over 50 who did experience chickenpox as a child, health professionals suggest they receive a shingles vaccine to prevent an outbreak of shingles.

For Further Information

Rosebloom, Ashley. *Shingles: Herpes Zoster Virus: Symptoms Treatment Causes Cures.* Printed by Amazon Digital Services, 2013.

Human Bites: The Mouth Has Dangerous Bacteria

- About 10 to 15 percent of human bite wounds become infected
- Human mouth has as many as 100 million organisms per milliliter, with as many as 190 different species
- The bacterium *Eikenella corrodens* is the most dangerous in the human mouth

In the mid-800s, Vikings from Norway captured the northern coast of present day Scotland, but not without a fight with the determined tribes that lived there. Sigurd the Powerful was the leader of the Viking conquest, and he went into battle against the Scottish tribes led by Máel Brigte, also known as "Máel Brigte the Bucktoothed." Sigurd killed Máel Brigte and severed his head. He attached the severed head to his saddle to show the Vikings their victory. As he was riding on rough roads, the buck teeth of the severed head scratched the leg of Sigurd. Several days later, he died from the bite of the dead man.

WHAT ARE HUMAN BITES?

Of all admissions to the emergency rooms, bite injuries represent about 1 percent. Human bites are the most common, after dog and cat bites. About 10 to 15 percent of these human bites become infected. This infection occurs because the flora of the human mouth is ridden with as many as 190 different species of organisms, some of them exceptionally dangerous.

In 1958, Dr. M. Eiken found there was a slow growing rod-shaped bacterium that did not grow in oxygen but preferred carbon dioxide. When he grew the bacteria in a medium called blood agar, he found this bacterium made pits in the agar. Later researchers named the bacterium after Dr. Eiken, *Eikenella corrodens.* In the body, this bacteria reproduces rapidly and may cause infection from just a small tooth cut. Other bacteria in the mouth may also cause infections.

There are two basic types of bite injuries: clenched-fist injuries and occlusive injuries.

Clenched-fist injury. These occur when a clenched or closed fist comes into contact with another individual's teeth (such as during a fight). Only a small tooth cut of 3 to 8 millimeters in length can introduce the bacteria.

Most of these types of injuries occur during fights, especially barroom brawls. The person may go to the emergency room where the attendant makes the mistake of suturing the laceration. This sets up the conditions for *Eikenella,* an anaerobe that thrives in the absence of oxygen. People with the wound may be fooled by its tiny size. These wounds are serious and require aggressive treatment. However, most people with these clenched-fist injuries do not even seek help until the infection is so far advanced as to cause serious damage.

Occlusive bites. These types of bites occur when there is sufficient force to break the skin. The muscles in the human jaw are some of the strongest in the body, and the sharp incisor teeth are capable of biting off an individual's finger, ear, or nose. These types of bites can lead to deep injury, crushing and tearing tissues, or to complete loss of an area of skin (evulsion). A famous case illustrating an occlusive bite occurred in 1997, when in a prize fight, boxer Mike Tyson bit off part of the ear of his opponent Evander Holyfield.

Both clench-fist and occlusive bites send bacteria into the wound. These microbes can be aerobes (ones that can live in an oxygenated environment) or they can be anaerobes (bacteria that grow when injected deeply into a wound where no air is present). The common aerobes are *Staphylococcus, Streptococcus*, and *Corynebacteria.* About 30 percent of infected bite wounds have the common bacteria *Staphylococcus aureus*. Anaerobes include species of *Bacteriodes, Fusobacteria, Prevotella,* and *Peptostreptococcus*. All these bacteria can cause infection.

Human bites may also transmit certain diseases, which can be life threatening. Hepatitis B is found in the saliva of 75 percent of infected patients. Less likely is the transmission of HIV, which appears to be relatively low.

WHAT ARE THE SIGNS AND SYMPTOMS?

Signs that a bite wound may be infected include redness, pain, warmth, swelling, and drainage of pus. If not treated promptly, localized infections may spread to other areas of the body and cause more serious symptoms, including blood poisoning (sepsis) and organ failure.

HOW IS IT DIAGNOSED?

Many people with human bites try to diagnosed and self-treat. However, any human bite injury should be seen by a health care professional. Even so, some doctors may not realize the severe nature of the organisms in the human mouth. A swab from the wound may be taken to identify which bacteria are present.

WHAT IS THE TREATMENT?

In addition to basic wound care, antibiotics will be given if infection is observed or suspected. If people seek help immediately, the prognosis of treatment with antibiotics is very good. However, those who seek help several weeks after the injury, when infection is obvious, may experience serious complications, including the loss of a limb or some type of permanent cosmetic damage. Prior to antibiotics, up to 20 percent of human bite victims lost their fingers.

For Further Information
"Human Bites." Medscape. http://emedicine.medscape.com/article/218901-overview.

Human Botfly: Tropical Vacationers Beware

- Known also as *Dermatobia hominis*; torsalo; and American warble fly
- Native to southeastern Mexico, Central America, and northern Argentina

- Flies attach eggs to a mosquito or other insects that land on human skin and deposit eggs
- Larvae hatch and bore into human skin, breathing through a small hole

Diane R. came into the emergency room (ER) complaining that she had bugs in her scalp. The doctor could find nothing. She came back the same day with the same complaint; again, the doctor found nothing. The next day she and her husband returned; he had seen an insect come out and then go back into a small hole on his wife's scalp. This time the doctor saw it too and worked to extract it. He admitted that he had never seen anything like this.

Diane had gone to Costa Rica and spent a night in the rainforest. There, unbeknownst to her, she had picked up the human botfly.

WHAT IS THE HUMAN BOTFLY?

Dematobia hominis is one of several species of flies that have human hosts. The name comes from Greek roots: *derma,* meaning "skin," *bio,* meaning "life," and from the Latin *hominis,* meaning "man." Several other species are parasites on cattle, deer, and other mammals. The common name is botfly. The botfly is endemic in certain tropical regions of Central and South America. It is especially prominent in the forest and jungle areas of Costa Rica and Belize.

The life cycle of this botfly is quite complex. The females do not deposit their eggs directly onto humans. After mating, adult females grab onto other bugs, such as mosquitoes (especially), ticks, or other biting flies. She holds the wings so the insect cannot escape and glues about 15 to 20 eggs onto the belly of the biting insect. Then, the insect finds a host for its own feeding, and when the eggs feel the warmth of the human body, they drop off the underside of the biting insect and hatch into larvae. The larvae then burrow into the skin either on their own or through the bite of the mosquito and create an air hole for breathing.

The larvae stay put. They do not migrate to other parts of the body but may move around under the skin, causing irritation and pain. The head of the larva grabs onto the host tissue e using two oral hooks for feeding. Curved spines located on the body help keep the larvae in place. The posterior end is located near the surface of the skin, and a hole enables the larvae to breathe and to excrete waste. The larvae goes through two molts and then enters a third stage in which it emerges and drops to the ground. The whole process takes between 14 and 30 days. Now it is an adult. It does not feed and lives only a short period of time, looking to reproduce and repeat the cycle.

WHAT ARE THE SIGNS AND SYMPTOMS?

Human botflies create telltale raised bumps in the skin with a small hole at the center. Those infested will feel sharp pains, as the larvae feed on living tissue.

HOW IS IT DIAGNOSED?

Diagnosis is very tricky. Because of their unfamiliarity with the human botfly, many health professionals in the United States have misdiagnosed it. Most commonly, it is mislabeled as an infected insect bite and antibiotics are prescribed, which do no good. A tentative diagnosis may be made if the person has traveled to an area where botflies are endemic and has a lump that does not heal. Finding the breathing hole, while difficult, is a telltale clue.

WHAT IS THE TREATMENT?

If the breathing hole is covered, the larvae will come out. Anything that will adequately cover the hole can be used: nail polish, tape, wax, vaseline or oil, for instance. These substances prevents air from reaching the larvae, and the partial asphyxiation will weaken them. Once the larvae have been weakened, they can then be grasped with tweezers or by applying pressure to both sides of the lump. Some folk remedies include putting a piece of meat over the hole to entice the larvae to come out and into the meat. Digging in the skin to try to get the larva out may cause it to burst or break apart and cause infection. It is best to have a physician remove the larvae.

To minimize the risk of botfly infestation, travelers should wear protective clothing and use insect repellents to minimize the risk of being bitten by a mosquito carrying botfly eggs.

For Further Information

Boggild, Andrea K., Jay S. Keystone, and Kevin C. Kain. August 2002. "Furuncular Myiasis: A Simple and Rapid Method for Extraction of Intact *Dermatobia hominis* Larvae." *Clinical Infectious Diseases* 35 (3): 336–338.

Leprosy: A Disease with a Past

- Name changed to Hansen's disease because of historical stigma of leprosy
- Prevalence in 2012: 189,018 cases in world; about 100 people are diagnosed with leprosy every year in the United States
- Chronic disease caused by slowly multiplying bacillus *Mycobacterium leprae*
- Disease affects skin, peripheral nerves, respiratory tract, and eyes

From early times, one disease was so feared that people isolated the affected individuals in colonies. At times, those with the disease were forced to wear special clothing and have bells that warned of their approach. Scientists know a lot more about the disease today, and that it is not as contagious as people once assumed. However, the mention of the name leprosy still evokes great fear.

WHAT IS LEPROSY?

Leprosy, also known as Hansen's disease, is a chronic infectious disease caused by the bacterium *Mycobacterium leprae*. The disease presents as skin sores, peripheral nerve damage, lung, and eye weakness, all of which get worse over time. The bacterium is slow growing, and it may take as long as 20 years for the symptoms to appear from the time the person was first exposed.

The word "leprosy" comes from the Latin word *Lepra*, meaning "scaly." One of the first noticeable symptoms is the effect on the skin.

In the past, people with leprosy were considered unclean and untouchable. Researchers believe that as early as 4,000 BCE, individuals had leprosy. The first known reference appeared in an Egyptian papyrus in 1,500 BCE. The Bible mentions leprosy as a special curse from God; lepers were left in colonies or as outcasts from society. References are also made in the writings of ancient China and India. People in these societies feared leprosy because they thought it was an incurable, mutilating, and very contagious disease. The Romans and the Crusaders, who went to areas of the Middle East, brought leprosy back to Europe.

There are three types of leprosy:

- *Tuberculoid.* This type is milder and less severe. The patches are flatter and the skin just feels numbs under the patches. This less contagious type is also called paucibacillary leprosy.
- *Lepromatous.* This severe form of the disease has widespread bumps and rashes, numbness, and all the above symptoms. The nose, kidneys, and male reproductive organs are affected. This more contagious type is also called multibacillary leprosy.
- *Borderline.* People with this type may have symptoms of both forms.

In 1873, Dr. Gerhard Armauer Hansen (1841–1912), a Norwegian scientist, discovered the bacterium that caused leprosy, *Mycobacterium leprae* or *M. leprae*. All members of the genus *Mycobacterium* are rod-shaped bacilli that are surrounded by tough waxy coats, making it very difficult to culture with regular laboratory procedures. However, they can be cultivated in the lab in animals such as chimpanzees, macaques, and armadillos. Tuberculosis is a member of the same family of Mycobacterium. The species name *leprae* is the one that Hansen isolated as the cause. Armadillos have been known to carry leprosy and are used in research today on Hansen's disease.

Although the organism was identified in the 19th century, patients were still encouraged or forced to live in colonies, even in the United States, until 1940s. Two leper colonies were located in the United States: one at Molokai in Hawaii, established by a priest known as Father Damien, who also had leprosy, and another at Carville, Louisiana. The facility at Carville has become a live-in treatment and research center. Currently, only about 11 people live there; the rest of the facility exists as a museum of leprosy and houses research facilities. There are still some mandatory colonies in India and China.

WHAT ARE THE SIGNS AND SYMPTOMS?

Leprosy is an unusual disease, because the person may have the condition for many years before symptoms appear. The term "incubation period" refers to the time there is first contact with the organism until the time symptoms of the disease begin to appear. Some people do not develop the symptoms for 20 years. This long incubation period makes it difficult to diagnose, and for doctors to determine exactly when the person came in contact with the causative agent.
Following are the symptoms and signs of the disease:

- Disfiguring skin sores that do not go away. The sores may appear as bumps or lumps and are lighter colored than the normal skin color.
- Peripheral nerve damage. The peripheral nerves are those that go to body extremities and are outside the central nervous system of the brain and spinal cord. This nerve damage causes loss of feeling in the arms and legs.
- Muscle weakness
- Affects the mucosal lining of the skin inside the nose
- Affects the eyes and may cause blindness

If left untreated, any of the forms can cause permanent damage to skin and limbs. In folklore, there are tales of the limbs actually falling off; but this does not happen as a direct result of leprosy. However, if untreated, secondary infections can cause tissue damage that can cause loss of fingers, toes, or serious deformity.

HOW IS IT DIAGNOSED?

Doctors and residents of the United States may be unaware of leprosy and its symptoms. There are many common symptoms with other conditions: runny nose, dry scalp, skin patches or lines, red skin, and loss of sensation in fingers and toes. When leprosy is suspected, the physician may order a skin biopsy or a skin scraping to check for the presence of the leprosy bacteria. The lepromin skin test can be used to tell the difference between the various forms.

WHAT IS THE TREATMENT?

The search for an effective treatment for leprosy also has a long history. In early years, the oil of the chaulmoogra nut was used, although the treatments were painful and of dubious benefit. In 1941, the sulfone drug promin was initiated at Carville, but these treatments were also painful. In the 1950s, dapsone became the treatment of choice, but the bacteria soon became resistant to this drug. In the 1970s, the first multidrug treatment, a regimen that combined dapsone, rifampicin, and clofazimine, was used. Anti-inflammatory drugs may also be given to reduce certain symptoms. Although treatment may take several months, leprosy is now considered curable.

For Further Information

Everest, Frank. *Leprosy: Quick Facts about This Misunderstood Disease.* Amazon Digital Services: Skin Diseases, Skin Disorders, and Skin Treatments, 2015.

Naegleria fowleri: Brain-Eating Amoeba

- An amoeba found in warm freshwater lakes and rivers
- Travels up the nose to the brain causing primary amoebic meningoencephalitis (PAM)
- Very rare: From 2003 to 2012, only 38 infections in the United States
- Fatality rate is greater than 95 percent

The summer is a great time to go to lakes, beaches, and waterparks, but it can be dangerous. In July, 2013, Kali Hardig, a 12-year-old girl from Arkansas, became very ill after a visit to a water park called Willow Springs in Little Rock. She was diagnosed with an unusual brain disease that she had contracted from the water in the park. She was treated with an experimental drug miltefosine. In addition, physicians reduced her body temperature to 93 degrees, a technique used to treat brain injury patients in order to preserve brain tissue. She is one of the first cases to survive the brain-eating amoeba.

In August 2013, Zachary Rehna, a 12-year-old Florida boy, was kneeboarding in a freshwater channel near his Miami home. He slept all the next day, a feat that caused his mother to take him to the hospital. The doctors diagnosed him with PAM. Doctors at Miami Children's Hospital treated the boy with the same treatment that had been performed the month before in Arkansas. As of early 2014, both children have survived and are still attending rehabilitation.

WHAT IS *NAEGLERIA FOWLERI*?

Naegleria is the genus name for a one-celled organism called an amoeba that lives in warm freshwater lakes, rivers, hot springs, and soil. Amoeba are the simplest of the protozoa or one-celled animals. Amoeba (plural) exist in three forms: one that has a flagella or whip-like structure, a cyst form that is inactive, and the trophozoites or feeding form.

Only one species, *N. fowleri,* is dangerous to humans. This microscopic organism in only about 8 to 14 micrometers wide, which in small in comparison to a human hair, which is about 40 to 50 micrometers wide. The feeding form exists in the warm waters of lakes, rivers, and lime pits, but it can also be found in poorly chlorinated swimming pools, hot springs, thermal runoffs from power plants, aquariums, poorly maintained hot water heaters, and soil. The amoeba is a thermophile and thrives in waters with temperatures of 115°F (46°C) or higher.

Most cases occur in southern or southwestern states, with over half found in Florida and Texas. However, during a very hot August in 2010, a child contracted the organism from a lake in Minnesota. A few cases have been contracted when individuals irrigated their sinuses with a device called a neti pot, an old yogi technique from India. The presence of the organism has been found also in in public water systems and pipes, including public drinking water systems. Amoeba do not live in salt water.

Two Australian scientists, M. Fowler and R. F. Carter, first described the organism in 1965. The amoeba was named for Fowler. The scientists named the infection caused by this amoeba "protozoan primary amoebic meningoencephalitis" (PAM) to distinguish it from other amoeba, such as *Entamoeba histolytica,* an amoeba that invades the human intestinal system. A study of the history of the disease revealed the first case of PAM probably occurred in Great Britain in 1909.

Although infections of this organism are rare, the potential of infection for those who are swimming in lakes and rivers, as well as other areas, is always present. Many popular tourist destinations include lakes and rivers. The high count of amoeba occurs in the months of July and August, which coincide with high tourist traffic.

N. fowleri enters the nose and then eats its way along the olfactory nerve, one of the seven cranial nerves that lead to the brain. As the amoeba feeds on brain tissue, the person experiences the symptoms of PAM, and eventually dies from infection.

WHAT ARE THE SIGNS AND SYMPTOMS?

When the person is exposed to the organism, it takes one to seven days for symptoms to appear. At first, the person begins to have changes in taste and smell, headache, fever, nausea, and vomiting. Then, other symptoms such as stiff neck, confusion, loss of balance, seizures, and hallucinations occur. The symptoms are similar to other kinds of meningitis. The disease progresses rapidly, with death usually occurring in about five days.

HOW IS IT DIAGNOSED?

Diagnosis is very difficult because the onset is sudden, and the person is not likely to realize that amoeba were in the water. The symptoms are similar to other diseases, so the delay in diagnosis can be fatal. Most cases are diagnosed at autopsy. In order to determine the presence of the amoebae, scientists can grow them on a number of laboratory media. Unfortunately, this finding may be too late for the patient.

WHAT IS THE TREATMENT?

Several drugs, such as amphotericin B have been effective *in vitro* (in a laboratory setting with cells cultured in a dish), but were not successful when given to patients. Treatments have combined several therapies, such as miltefosine and induced hypothermia, with limited but promising success.

At present, there is no routine or rapid test for *N. Fowleri* in the water. Anyone who swims in the water should assume the presence of this common amoeba.

The CDC recommends that people not swim in fresh water lakes when the temperature is high and the water is low. The swimmer should avoid stirring up the sediment when wading in lakes. Use of nose clips when swimming is also advised. People can avoid the organism by avoiding risky behaviors, such as diving or jumping into the water, holding the head under water, or engaging in activities that cause water to go up the nose. Also, if you are irrigating your sinuses with a neti pot, be sure to use distilled or sterilized water, not tap water.

For Further Information

"*Naegleria fowleri*—Primary Amebic Meningoencephalitis (PAM)." Centers for Disease Control and Prevention. http://www.cdc.gov/parasites/naegleria/.

Necrotizing Fasciitis: The Flesh-Eating Disease

- Caused by several kinds of bacteria
- About 500–1500 cases per year in the United States
- 20 percent mortality rate
- Bacteria do not "eat" flesh but emit toxins that destroy tissue

In April 2012, Aimee Copeland, an energetic University of Georgia graduate student, was ziplining across the Little Tallapoosa River when she fell into the river. She sustained a deep cut in her leg that did not seem to heal. When her leg began to turn black, she went to the doctor and began a long bout with necrotizing fasciitis. The surgeons eventually had to amputate a leg, one foot, and both hands. She received two hands that cost $100,000 each, as well as artificial limbs, with which she learned to walk. Aimee thinks she is lucky to be alive because this condition can be fatal.

WHAT IS NECROTIZING FASCIITIS?

Necrotizing fasciitis (NF), sometimes referred to as flesh-eating disease, is a bacterial infection that affects the body's soft tissue. Several kinds of bacteria can cause the disorder. The condition is usually not common in healthy people like Aimee, but more often affects those with compromised immune systems. However, it is definitely unpredictable. If left untreated or ignored, the condition is fatal.

The name "necrotizing fasciitis" literally means "decaying infection of the fascia." The fascia are flat layers of connective bands that surround muscles, nerves, fat, and blood vessels. They are located in the deep layers of subcutaneous tissues. The bacteria enter through an opening in the skin. The opening can be something as simple as a paper cut, a staple puncture, a blister, or bruise; the bacteria can also enter through a major trauma or surgery. Sometimes, the place of entry may not be known.

Dr. B. Wilson, writing in a 1952 issue of *American Surgery*, first described the necrosis of underlying subcutaneous tissue and called it necrotizing fasciitis. The name flesh-eating bacteria, so popular in the press, is really a misnomer. The bacteria do not eat the flash but emit toxins that destroy the tissues.

Several types of bacteria may be involved. The one most common is Group A Streptococcus (*S. pyogenes*). Other bacteria include *Staphylococcus aureus, Clostridium perfringens, Bacteroides fragilis,* and *Aeromonas hydrophila*. A person with NF may have a number of different organisms, which is designated Type I or polymicrobial; the person may have one kind, which is designated Type II or monomicrobial. Most cases are Type I. However, since 2001, another monomicrobial form has been caused by methicillin-resistant *Staphylococcus aureus* or MRSA.

NF is one of the conditions tracked by the Centers for Disease Control and Prevention (CDC), and must be reported to the CDC.

WHAT ARE THE SIGNS AND SYMPTOMS?

The sudden onset may be confusing because it may resemble other illnesses. The symptoms most common at the beginning are pain or soreness that is similar to a pulled muscle. Then, the person may develop fever, chills, or vomiting, which also occur in many conditions. Because these symptoms are similar to some common conditions, an individual may delay getting help.

Early symptoms begin within 24 hours, and the pain occurs in the place where the bacteria have entered. Within three to four days, the limb begins to swell and develops a purplish rash. The limb may have a large, dark raised area that develops blisters that ooze with dark fluid. At this point, the wound looks like the flesh is being destroyed and becomes bluish-white with a mottled appearance. Blood pressure drops, and the body goes into shock in response to the toxins given off by the bacteria. The person becomes extremely weak and may fall unconscious. Death occurs if the person is not treated.

HOW IS IT DIAGNOSED?

The diagnosis is not simple. Growing of the responsible bacteria may take time. However, with severe symptoms, treatment may begin before a definitive diagnosis is made.

HOW IS IT TREATED?

Antibiotics should be started as soon as the condition is suspected. The affected tissue is removed, a process called debridement. Medications must be given to raise blood pressure, and a new medicine called intravenous immunoglobulin (IVIG) may be used. Sometimes the person is treated in a hyperbaric chamber. This chamber in which the atmospheric pressure is increased has been used to treat various deep wounds that do not respond to other treatments. The person will probably have scars that require skin grafting. Some people may have to have the affected limb amputated in order to stop the spread of the bacteria.

CASE HISTORY: MARY RYAN'S ORDEAL

Mary, a native of Ireland, was living in Central Florida in a town north of Orlando. Although she had had heart bypass sugary only a year earlier, she asked for a liposuction procedure, because she was concerned about the collection of fat in her abdomen. The doctor at the clinic considered her fit for the procedure, which she underwent on December 19, 2012. However, she later complained of nausea and pain in her abdomen, and was prescribed pain medications. Mary did not go to the doctor for her scheduled checkup, because she was too nauseous. However, ignoring the pain and nausea, she decided to spend Christmas in Ireland, and did not bother to take her antibiotics.

When she arrived in Ireland, she went to bed immediately at her son's home, and her son, who was unaware of her surgery, was shocked to see her swollen, bruised, and battered abdomen. She was taken to Cork University Hospital, and despite treatment with high doses of antibiotics and surgical procedures that removed all deteriorating skin from her stomach, she deteriorated rapidly. The aggressive necrotizing fasciitis had spread too rapidly, causing her kidneys to shut down. She died on December 29.

For Further Information

Roemmele, Jacqueline A. *Surviving the Flesh-Eating Bacteria: Understanding, Preventing, Treating, and Living with Necrotizing Fasciitis.* New York: Avery, 2000.

Norovirus: Scourge of the Cruise Ship

- 19 to 21 million infections in the United States each year, including 570 to 800 deaths
- Highly contagious virus, transmitted especially in enclosed areas such as cruise ships
- Only need a few virus particles to be affected
- Some individuals appear to have genetic immunity to the virus

In February 2014, 114 passengers and six crew members on a cruise ship started vomiting, experienced diarrhea, and became extremely ill. Only a month before, 600 people sailing on a Caribbean cruise had had similar symptoms. The cause of the illness was traced to the norovirus. A passenger brings the virus onto the ship, and with so many people living in close quarters, the illness spreads rapidly. Although cruise ships are often blamed, many other places have experienced the spread of the virus, such as elementary schools and day care facilities.

WHAT IS NOROVIRUS?

Norovirus is a highly contagious infection characterized by nausea, vomiting, diarrhea, and abdominal cramping. No vaccine prevents it, and no drugs treat it. Most people get better after one to three days of dealing with the symptoms. It can spread rapidly through an enclosed place like a cruise ship. This virus is different from many other viruses, in that only a small amount of the virus can lead to infection.

The virus was originally known as the Norwalk virus, named after the town of Norwalk, Ohio, where the first case emerged among schoolchildren at Bronson Elementary School in November 1968. The name Norwalk virus was given in 1972 and later shortened to norovirus, after being identified as the cause of several severe outbreaks on cruise ships. There are several different strains of the virus, but all have similar symptoms. The common name "stomach flu" is a misnomer; norovirus is not related to influenza. The United Kingdom has an interesting name for the virus; it is called winter vomiting bug. This bug spreads during cold weather when people are shut up in close quarters. In 2012, a new strain called GII.4 Sydney infected people in many countries, and is now the leading cause of most current outbreaks.

PROTECT YOURSELF AND OTHERS FROM NOROVIRUS

1. Wash your hands thoroughly with soap and water after going to the bathroom, and especially before preparing food. This does not mean just sticking one hand under the water. Use the old trick taught to children: Lather with soap as long as it will take to sing the lines of "Happy Birthday to You," then rinse and dry with a clean towel. Alcohol-based sanitizers can reduce germs, but do not take the place of soap and water.
2. Do not prepare food while infected. Experts tell us you can infect others before you have symptoms and for three days or longer afterwards.
3. Clean and disinfect contaminated surfaces using a bleach-based cleanser. When you are on a cruise ship, airplane, or other areas with large numbers of people in an enclosed area, take care not to touch counters and other areas unnecessarily.
4. Wash fruits and vegetables well with running water. Cook shellfish thoroughly.
5. Wash laundry thoroughly. Handle any soiled items carefully—wear rubber gloves if possible. Wash with detergent with the maximum cycle and machine dry.

Norovirus affects people of all ages, and is the most common stomach and intestinal virus. It is usually spread through aerosol droplets from a contaminated individual, but it can also be transmitted through contaminated food or water. This is especially true for raw fruits and vegetables, and raw or undercooked oysters. The virus can also be picked up just by touching contaminated surfaces. Fewer than 20 virus particles can cause an infection; some researchers say as few as five particles is sufficient. To acquire infection from most viruses, the person needs to be exposed to 100 or more individual virions. These viruses are hardy. They can survive extreme temperatures in water and on hard surfaces for weeks. They have been found to contaminate fabrics for over 12 days, and may survive in contaminated water for years.

Interestingly, some individuals may have partial or complete resistance to certain strains of norovirus. These individuals, known as "non-secretors," do not have a functioning copy of the FUT2 gene, which codes for the production of particular enzymes on the surface of certain body cells. These enzymes are necessary for infection by the most common strain of norovirus. These individuals may still be susceptible to other strains of norovirus, as well as other viruses that may cause gastroenteritis.

WHAT ARE THE SIGNS AND SYMPTOMS?

Noroviruses are actually a group of viruses that cause gastrointestinal infections. They are characterized by forceful vomiting, nausea, watery diarrhea, and terrible abdominal pain. Other symptoms may also be present, such as weakness, headache, low-grade fever, and general lethargy. Symptoms usually resolve in one to three days. Complications may arise; most notably dehydration as a result of profuse vomiting and diarrhea. The very young, the elderly, and those with compromised immune systems are most at risk.

HOW IS IT DIAGNOSED?

The virus can be identified through routine assays of polymerase chain reaction (PCR), which can detect as few as 10 virus particles. The virus itself is very simple. It is a single strand of RNA and does not have an outside containing envelope. Diagnosis, however, is usually made based on a patient's symptoms and whether or not a general outbreak is suspected. In most cases, individuals who suspect that they have norovirus do not seek medical attention, and simply "ride it out."

WHAT IS THE TREATMENT?

The disease usually limits itself to one to three miserable days. People with the symptoms should try to stay away from others. There is no treatment for the virus itself, although treatment of the symptoms may provide some relief. It is especially important to stay hydrated. Surfaces need to be treated with chlorine-based disinfectants, but the virus is less susceptible to alcohols and detergents.

For Further Information

Stone, Carolyn. *Norovirus: How to Stay Safe*. New York: Eternal Spring Books, 2014.

Rocky Mountain Spotted Fever: Where Ticks Are

- Prevalence: About 800 cases reported each year in the United States
- Caused by *Rickettsia rickettsii*, a small bacteria
- Produces a telltale rash in 90 percent of cases
- Originally found in the Rocky Mountains, but now reported throughout the continental United States, Mexico, Canada, and South America

In 1947, the movie *Driftwood* brought attention to Rocky Mountain spotted fever. An orphan named Jenny finds a collie that had escaped from a wrecked plane in the Rocky Mountains. The dog has a note on his collar, saying he was to be used to develop an experimental vaccine for tick fever. Both the dog and little girl are adopted by a doctor who is doing research on the fever and who believes the fever is carried by ticks. However, the leaders of the town do not like his ideas, and one night, they destroy his laboratory. Infested ticks are then released into the community. The people of the town then beg for a cure for Rocky Mountain spotted fever.

WHAT IS ROCKY MOUNTAIN SPOTTED FEVER?

Rocky Mountain spotted fever (RMSF) is a serious disease carried by ticks. The ticks carry a very small bacteria called *rickettsia*. When the person is bitten by the tick, the bacteria causes serious damage to the cells lining the blood vessels. Spots develop where the blood vessels break, which gave the condition the name "spotted fever." If not treated, the condition can be lethal.

Actually, the name "Rocky Mountain spotted fever" is a misnomer. It was originally recognized in the Rocky Mountains, but since the 1930s it has also been found throughout the United States, especially in the southern states, as well as in Canada and in Central and South America.

This condition is the most lethal of all rickettsial diseases, and is probably more common than once thought. There are two ticks that carry the disease: the American dog tick (*Dermacentor variabilis)* and the Rocky Mountain wood tick (*Dermacentor andersoni*). Many people have pets that could possibly have ticks, or hike and camp in areas with ticks.

WHAT ARE THE SIGNS AND SYMPTOMS?

The tick bites, but many people will not even realize it, because there is no pain. But in two to 14 days, the person will develop a sudden onset of fever and headache, symptoms that are similar to other conditions and may be treated at home with over-the-counter medications. The person may then experience nausea, vomiting, muscle pain, lack of appetite, and abdominal pain that mimics appendicitis. All these are similar to other conditions.

However, the main symptom is rash, which may occur in 90 percent of cases. In a classic case, the rash develops about two to five days after the onset of fever, and appears as small, pink spots on the wrists, forearms, ankles, trunk, and soles of the feet. Then the rash may go from red to purple, a sign of severe progression of the disease. The rash may not be present in about 10 percent of patients with the infection.

The infection carried by the tick affects blood vessels, tissues, and organs throughout the body. The lungs, spinal cord, heart, liver, and kidneys are affected. The linings of the vessels of the organs rupture. This causes a symptom known as petechiae, which occurs from bleeding through the skin. In some severe cases, the loss of blood supply to body parts may cause injury to the organ and dysfunction. People with severe infection may require hospitalization, and have long-term health problems. Although RMSF is serious, today the mortality rate is less than 1 percent.

HOW IS IT DIAGNOSED?

RMSF is very difficult to diagnose in the early stages. Younger patients may have the rash earlier than older patients. For those with no rash, it is extremely easy to misdiagnose. Laboratory tests may indicate elevated liver enzyme levels, thrombocytopenia, and low sodium (hyponatremia). If RMSF is suspected, blood tests can be run to check for the presence of the rickettsia bacteria.

WHAT IS THE TREATMENT?

Treatment with doxycycline, a tetracycline antibiotic, should be started immediately after diagnosis. The first line of treatment is the most effective if started within five days of symptoms. If treatment is delayed and other organs are affected, a specialist must be called in to treat those conditions.

For anyone going outside into areas where ticks may be present, all precautions should be taken. Always use a preventive insecticide that has DEET or another chemical that targets ticks and insects. Wear long pants and sleeves to prevent ticks from attaching themselves and biting. Consider spraying permethrin, a powerful insecticide, on clothes and camping gear to help repel ticks. Also, pets should be given special treatments that protect them from ticks and fleas.

For Further Information
Walker, David H. *Rocky Mountain Spotted Fever.* New York: Chelsea House, 2007.

Valley Fever: Coccidioidomycosis

- More than 20,000 cases reported each year in the United States, but many more likely go undiagnosed
- Fungal infection caused by coccidioides
- Found in soil of the Southwest; endemic in parts of Arizona, California, Nevada, New Mexico, Texas, Utah, and northern Mexico
- Most cases end on their own, but some cause serious problems

Dr. Sharon Nagami, a California infectious disease specialist and author, tells of going to the funeral of a patient named Roger on a hot August afternoon. She had worked so hard to save him. But she had been defeated by a tiny fungus. She described how the strong winds that blow in Southern California between Thanksgiving and Christmas bring in tiny spores that take up residence in lungs of people in the area. She had gone to only four funerals in her practice, and two were young men with cocci. Cocci is the short name given to Coccidioidomycosis, known also as Valley fever, and a disease that is largely unknown except to those living in the Southwestern United States.

WHAT IS VALLEY FEVER?

Valley fever is a fungal infection caused by *Coccidioides immitis*. The fungi inhabit the soil and grow mycelium, a mass of branching thread-like structures, until the rains come. Then, they break off into smaller airborne spores, called arthroconidia. Something then comes to disturb them. Farming, construction, or just a strong wind can pick up the dust that has the fungi spores in it, and spread the tiny spores everywhere across the Southwest. They have even been found as far north as Washington State. The condition is not contagious from one person to another, but is transferred through the wind.

Anyone can get Valley fever, including children. It is most common among older adults. With more people, especially retirees, now moving to the Sun Belt states of Arizona, New Mexico, and Nevada, more serious cases are expected. In addition to humans, dogs, cats, and most mammals can also get Valley fever.

WHAT ARE THE SIGNS AND SYMPTOMS?

About 40 percent of cases begin like the flu, with fever, cough, headaches, chest pain, muscle pain, fatigue, and joint pain. A red spotty rash may be a telltale sign that it is not just flu. The red rash appears as painful, raised red bumps on the lower extremities and on chest, arms, and back. It may form a blister-like necklace, especially in women. Certain ethnic groups appear to be more at risk. Those groups at risk include those of Filipino, African, Native American, Hispanic, and Asian backgrounds. Those who have some type of immune system problems are also more susceptible.

Three basic forms of the condition exist: acute, chronic, and disseminated.

- *Acute coccidioidomycosis.* This type has flu-like symptoms and rash. The symptoms can persist for several months, with fatigue and joint pain lasting much longer. The health of the individual and the number of spores inhaled seems to determine the severity.
- *Chronic coccidioidomycosis.* The symptoms do not go away, and may progress to a form of pneumonia. The person will experience low-grade fever, weight loss, cough, chest pain, blood-tinged sputum (matter coughed up), and nodules in the lungs.
- *Disseminated coccidioidomycosis.* This form goes from the lungs to other parts of the body, which can include skin, bones, liver, brain, heart, and

the meninges, the covering of the brain and spinal cord. These very serious conditions can lead to death.

HOW IS IT DIAGNOSED?

Diagnosis may be difficult. Nodules on the X-ray may lead the doctor to incorrectly suspect lung cancer. Doctors outside of the Southwest may be unfamiliar with Valley fever, so if one becomes ill after traveling to the Southwest, it is wise to let the doctor know. The fungus can be detected in body fluids. It is commonly misdiagnosed as pneumonia or cancer.

WHAT IS THE TREATMENT?

Treating the symptoms and making the person comfortable is extremely important. Antifungal treatment with intravenous amphotericin B can be very painful, and used only with those who are immunosuppressed. Other drugs are being tested.

For those who live in the area, the best advice is prevention by avoiding airborne dust or dirt, but this is not easy and not certain. People may be advised to wear face masks during the windy seasons.

For Further Information

Rundbaken, Craig. *Valley Fever Silent Epidemic: The Common, Often Misdiagnosed Desert Ailment*. Sun City West, AZ: Craig Rundbaken, 2014.

West Nile Virus: From Birds to Mosquitoes to Humans

- A virus carried from infected birds to mosquitoes to humans
- Over 1,000 cases reported to the Centers for Disease Control and Prevention to date
- Texas is the hardest-hit state in the United States
- 70–80 percent of people who become infected do not develop symptoms

Yellow fever had been a threat to people through the tropical and subtropical world since the 1600s. The search for the virus was important to the economy and well-being of several nations, so modern scientists sought to identify this virus as soon as possible. In 1937, while looking for the yellow fever virus, a new virus was isolated from a 37-year-old woman in Omogo in the West Nile district of Uganda. The same virus was seen in Egypt in 1942, in India in 1953, and later in other places in the world. However, it was not seen in the Western Hemisphere until 1999. The U.S. outbreak started in College Point, Queens in New York City, and soon spread to other states. As of August 2012, the Centers for Disease Control and Prevention (CDC) has confirmed 1,118 cases of West Nile virus, with cases in 47 states.

WHAT IS WEST NILE VIRUS?

West Nile virus (WNV) is capable of causing disease in humans, and appears to be potentially anywhere. The person first begins to experience flu-like symptoms, which are similar to the beginning of many other diseases. However, in older adults, very young children, or those with compromised immune systems, more serious disorders may develop that affect the brain and spinal cord. The virus is spread to people through mosquitoes, which acquire the virus from birds.

The virus is carried by female *Culex pipiens* mosquitoes. Female mosquitoes are the only ones that feed on blood. The primary host that serves as a reservoir are birds, especially passerines (songbirds). In addition to humans, WNV also affects other mammals, alligators and crocodiles, and amphibians. It is not spread by person-to-person contact.

WHAT ARE THE SIGNS AND SYMPTOMS?

The incubation time from infection to symptoms onset is typically between two to 15 days. Approximately 70–80 percent of persons who become infected do not experience any noticeable symptoms. West Nile fever occurs in 20 percent of cases. The person has fever and flu-like symptoms, such as chills, excessive sweating, joint pain, and some gastrointestinal problems. Most people with this type recover completely. Severe symptoms appear in less than 1 percent of cases. People develop neurological illness including encephalitis (inflammation of the brain) or meningitis (inflammation of the covering of the brain). In addition to fever and headache, the person may have neck stiffness, disorientation, coma, seizures, tremors, or paralysis. Death may also occur.

HOW IS IT DIAGNOSED?

A number of diseases have similar symptoms, at least in the beginning. Symptoms and a history of mosquito bites would be included in a preliminary diagnosis. Blood or cerebrospinal fluid tests will be administered if WNV is suspected. If antibodies are present and certain proteins are elevated, the disease can be confirmed. The US Food and Drug Administration (FDA) has approved WNV IgM ELISA test kits for use in patients who have the neurological symptoms.

WHAT IS THE TREATMENT?

There is no vaccine, nor any specific antiviral treatment for the infection. The treatment is supportive, including treating fever and other symptoms.

Prevention is still the best treatment. Individuals are advised to rid their property of places where mosquitoes breed, and to use insect repellent when going out of doors.

For Further Information

Abramovitz, Melissa. *West Nile Virus*. San Diego, CA: Lucent Books, 2013.

PART V

UNUSUAL DISEASES AND DISORDERS WITH OTHER OR UNEXPLAINED ORIGINS

WHAT YOU SHOULD KNOW ABOUT DISEASES AND DISORDERS WITH OTHER OR UNEXPLAINED ORIGINS

Most of these disorders were chosen because the cause is unknown or debatable. For example, no one knows why a person who has autism or some other mental disability may be able to calculate complex formulas, or be able to memorize books like Gibbon's *The Decline and Fall of the Roman Empire.*

Even in the day of advanced medicine and technology, there are many disorders and conditions that are have not been explained or understood. Medical researchers are making the effort to understand and treat these diseases. Research is complicated and expensive. Some doctors spend their entire professional lives studying one disease and then come away with more questions than answers.

Perhaps, one of the most puzzling conditions presented here are autoimmune diseases. Although the disorders may be recognized as autoimmune, the chemical pathways as to how the disorder begins or follows are still a mystery. The condition Anti-NMDA receptor encephalitis (AE) occurs when the immune system starts to attack the brain. Although scientists can describe the results, the reasons for such a complex disease are not known. The book *Brain on Fire: My Month of Madness* describes the ordeal of Susannah Cahalan, and how no one could figure out what her problem was. The book recounts how neurologist Souhel Najjar recognized her symptoms as belonging to a newly discovered autoimmune disorder, which had probably been around for centuries, when the afflicted persons would have been considered mad.

Several allergy conditions are presented. Most unusual is an allergy to water (aquagenic urticaria) or to certain foods that may interact with pollens (oral allergy syndrome or OAS).

One of the disorders, Morgellons syndrome, is hotly debated as a disorder. However, the people who have the symptoms declare that it exists.

The 22 disorders in this section do not fit neatly into genetic, mental, infectious, or environmental disorders categories. Some of them may cross over, and have some of the elements of one or the other, but still do not completely fit the pattern.

For Further Information

Asherson, Ronald, ed. *Handbook of Systemic Autoimmune Diseases* series. Amsterdam, Netherlands: Elsevier Science.

Anti-NMDA Receptor Encephalitis: When the Body Turns Against the Brain

- Prevalence: Unknown, but estimates suggest that 1 percent of encephalitis cases thought to be of unknown origin are AE
- Body's immune system attacks the brain
- Neuropsychiatric symptoms are prominent
- May be related to a type of tumor called a teratoma

An autoimmune disease occurs when the body has an inappropriate response against substances or tissues that are normally present in the body. The body actually turns against itself and makes antibodies. The word "encephalitis" is made of two Greek root words: *encephal* meaning "brain" and *itis* meaning "inflammation of."

WHAT IS ANTI-NMDA RECEPTOR ENCEPHALITIS?

Anti-NMDA receptor encephalitis (AE) is a condition in which the body's own immune system attacks the brain. Once considered to be very rare, more and more cases of AE are diagnosed as the condition becomes better known. Currently about 13 different antibodies are suspected, but only one Anti-NMDA receptor autoimmune encephalitis has a commercial test. With AE, a variety of neuropsychiatric symptoms may appear, and the disease can mimic other disorders. It may be or may not be connected with an ovarian teratoma.

First, let's look at the brain structure and neurons. Messages in the brain are carried by neurons and passed from one neuron to another across a gap called the synapse. Receptors on the neurons act to receive the messages. A receptor called N-methyl-D-aspartate (also known as NMDAR) is the primary device that controls for movement across the synapse and for memory function. The proper functioning of this receptor is essential for good brain functioning. The prefix "anti" means against. An antibody is a large Y-shaped protein produced by B-Cells that are used by the immune system to identify and neutralize foreign objects, such as bacteria or viruses. In this disease, the antibody is produced against the N-methyl-D-aspartate receptor.

AE was completely unknown until Dr. Josep Dalmau at University of Pennsylvania Medical School and a team of researchers wrote about anti-N-Methyl-D-Aspartate receptor encephalitis in a 2005 journal article in *The Lancet Neurology*. The condition they described was mostly associated with tumors of the ovaries; they referred to this as a paraneoplastic syndrome, which means it occurs in conjunction with a neoplasm or tumor.

A solid clue is the presence of a tumor called a teratoma. A teratoma is just as strange as its name—from the Greek *teratos* meaning "monster" and *oma* meaning "tumor." A teratoma is like something out of science fiction. However, these monstrosities have a long medical history. In 1658, one was found sprouting hair; they were given the name teratoma in 1863 when one was found in the mother's uterus that had hair, fatty tissue, teeth, and cartilage. It reminded the observer of a strange monstrous, disorganized embryo. In the 1899 edition of *Gray's Anatomy*, the text used by medical students, there was a chapter that dealt with teratology, the study of monsters. This chapter dealt with fetuses that were thought to have been marked as animals and monsters with no arranged bodies, but different body parts such as hair and teeth. In the past, teratomas were considered to be the result of witchcraft or dealings with the devil. Today they are looked upon as strange but benign.

However, it may be the presence of such tissues that generate the antibodies that then pass the blood-brain barrier and get into the brain. The blood-brain barrier ensures that most substances in the bloodstream meet a barrier before entering the brain. That is why treating brain disorders with medications is very difficult. Medications, which are generally large molecules, cannot get past the blood vessels that lead into the brain. These antibodies can get through the blood-brain barrier, because they have been generated in the nerve tissue present in the teratoma; there they can cause inflammation of the brain, or encephalitis.

WHAT ARE THE SIGNS AND SYMPTOMS?

With this disease the person can have a range of neuropsychiatric systems. Several symptoms mimic other neuropsychiatric disorders. Following are several of the symptoms:

- The condition may start with flu-like symptoms, such as fever, headache.
- Parts of the body became weak or numb.
- Balance is lost; speech is slurred.
- Cognitive and memory impairment occurs.
- The person develops dyskinesia, or erratic movements and seizures. The consciousness level may vary from unresponsiveness to coma.
- Person has an unexplained mixture of neuropsychiatric symptoms.

HOW IS IT DIAGNOSED?

A quick diagnosis and quick treatment is essential for a good recovery, but because the symptoms resemble other conditions, it is often misdiagnosed. The person may also have an MRI, which will show brain inflammation, and an electroencephalogram (EEG), which shows brain activity. One of the first clues is the presence of the teratoma, although all cases may not have the tumor.

A commercially available test that tests for the antibody is available at Athena Diagnostics or Mayo Clinic.

WHAT IS THE TREATMENT?

Treatments are broken down into first-line (initial) treatments and second-line treatments. Following are the most common primary treatments:

- Remove the teratoma that could be triggering the autoimmune response.
- Give the patient anti-inflammatory drugs such as steroids.
- Use a procedure known as plasmaphoresis to remove the antibodies from the blood.
- Treat with intravenous immunoglobulin (IVIG), a substance that may replace the binding sites where the antibodies attach to neurons.

CASE HISTORY: THE STORY OF SUSANNAH CAHALAN

Susannah Cahalan and her father kept notes of the impressions and descriptions of a 24-year-old who had anti-N-methyl-D-aspartate receptor encephalitis. They then converted their notes into a book, *Brain on Fire: My Month of Madness.*

Susannah recounts how she was at her desk at the *New York Post*, where she had landed a job as a reporter, when she noticed that something just did not feel right. After she completed an interview, she started crying hysterically for no reason at all, then suddenly brushed it off as if nothing had happened. She began to doubt herself, and eventually ended up in the office of a neurologist who did a number of tests. Nothing was wrong, he said. Maybe it is mono, or just a virus.

Later, she was watching television with her boyfriend, and suddenly she started grinding her teeth and biting her tongue, then passed out. That was the last thing she remembered, for a month after that.

Her actions became bizarre, and her paranoid delusions worsened. She imagined her father had murdered his wife. On the ride to the neurologist, she tried to jump out of the car as she screamed hysterically. She was admitted to the epilepsy ward at New York University Langone Medical Center. As the days passed, there were no answers as to what was happening to her.

Then doctors told her parents that there may be one last chance. A Syrian-born neurologist at the NYU hospital, Dr. Souhel Najjar, had been doing some experimental studies on a person's own antibodies attacking the brain. When the family met him, their confidence was boosted immediately. He gave Susannah a paper and told her to draw a clock. When she finished she had created a face of a clock with all the numbers on the right side and none on the left side. He now had some clue as to what was happening; it was some type of autoimmune encephalitis. He sent blood and spinal fluid to Dr. Josep Dalmau at the University of Pennsylvania Hospital to see if the rare antibodies were present. It was found that yes, there they were. Najjar started the treatments immediately: first, the intravenous immunoglobulin to reduce inflammation, then high levels of steroids. He then brought in the plasmapheresis machine to flush out the harmful antibodies.

Six months later, Susannah was back at work and back at home. When she thumbs through the pages of her father's notes, she marvels at the lost month of her life, and feels that she is reading about some stranger—not herself.

Following are the most common second-line treatments:

- Administer rituximab, an antibody injection that enables the immune system to destroy certain cells that create antibodies; this powerful medicine may have several adverse side effects.
- Administer CellCept, an oral immunosuppressant that was originally given to organ transplant patients. CellCept disrupts the formation of DNA in certain immune cells that are connected with autoimmune disorders. Like other strong treatments, it has side effects.
- Administer Cytoxan, a chemotherapy drug available in tablet or injectable form, which works to slow growth of certain immune cells.

For Further Information
Cahalan, Susannah. *Brain on Fire: My Month of Madness.* New York: Free Press, 2012.

Aquagenic Urticaria: Allergic to Water

- Very rare: Fewer than 100 cases reported in the literature
- Contact with water produces blisters and other signs of allergic reaction
- Underlying cause is unknown
- Treated with a variety of strategies

Water is a substance that makes up 70 percent of the earth and about 60 percent of the human body. It is essential for life, but some people can't take it. After Michaela Dutton, 21, had her first child, she noted red and white blisters after she took a bath. The dermatologist said that she had an allergy to water. She could only take very, very short showers, be vigilant when going outside for fear of rain, and take care when holding her son, because she is allergic to tears.

WHAT IS AQUAGENIC URTICARIA?

Aquagenic urticaria (AU) is a condition that occurs when the afflicted person comes into contact with water of any kind. The word "aquagenic" comes from two Latin words: *aqua,* meaning "water" and *gen* meaning "caused by"; urticaria is a term used by dermatologists to mean an itchy rash with raised areas, surrounded by redness. The condition is sometimes referred to in simplistic terms as "water allergy," but this is a misnomer. An allergic reaction occurs when histamine, a compound in the body, is released in response to allergens or inflammation; with an allergic reaction, histamine responses are at play. In this condition, none of this histamine reaction is present.

W. B. Shelley and T. M. Rawnsley reported the first cases of aquagenic urticaria in the 1964 *Journal of the American Medical Association*. They first described a 19-year-old man who had a terrible three-year history of small pinpoint-raised rashes on his shoulders, trunk, arms, abdomen, and back. Whenever the man took a shower or bath, this rash appeared within 10 to 20 minutes of the time when the water hit his skin; intense itching accompanied the rash. His rash lasted from 20 to 40 minutes, then went away on its own. He had no history of allergies, and the condition appeared when he came into contact with water.

Shelley and Rawnsley also reported about a four-year-old boy who had a similar condition, and who developed small pinpoints of wheals after contact with water. The episodes were documented for about a year, and like the older boy, he had no history of allergies.

Exposure to water is the problem. The condition may develop any place where water has touched the body. This could include bathing, swimming, or just walking in the rain. A person may react to his or her own perspiration or even tears. The rash develops from one to 15 minutes after exposure, and can lead to the painful lesions within 10 to 20 minutes. Some doctors surmise that the natural ions in the water along with additives such as chlorine may cause the problem. The temperature of the water does not appear to make a difference in the reaction.

Some other conditions are related to aquagenic urticaria. A person who is lactose intolerant may have a tendency. Other diseases, including HIV infections, Bernard–Soulier syndrome, and cholinergic urticaria appear to have a correlation. A possible familial pattern may also exist, which can be traced to its location on chromosome 2Q21. One group of researchers has suggested that the stratum corneum (the tough outer layer of the skin) or the sebum, the oily secretion of the sebaceous glands, generates a toxic compound that interacts with water. However, the cause is generally accepted as unknown.

WHAT ARE THE SIGNS AND SYMPTOMS?

The skin of people with aquagenic urticaria may respond to any type of water. Wheals, hives, and redness appear. Wheals are raised areas that may appear white but are surrounded by red areas and accompanied by itching. The condition may be quite painful. Someone with a severe case may react to drinking water and have difficulty swallowing, wheezing, or other respiratory conditions. For example, Rachel, 26, who lives in London where there is lots of rain, is so allergic to water that only one drop of rain will cause her to break out. Even saliva from the kisses of her fiancé causes a rash. However, some people have found their sensitivity decreases as they get older.

HOW IS IT DIAGNOSED?

After a medical history is taken, the person may be subjected to a water treatment test, which is applied to the upper body for 30 minutes. Distilled, tap, and saline (salt water) are used in the patches. The lesions are then inspected for the root cause of the problem.

WHAT IS THE TREATMENT?

A variety of actions can be used, none of which have been extremely effective. Most of the treatments are palliative. They seek to comfort the patient and are actually not a cure for the condition. Following are some of the suggested treatments:

- **Topical corticosteroids.** The benefits of applying steroids have not been established but may help some cases.
- **Epinephrine.** This compound is used to treat allergies, but some have tried using it to affect the skin rash.
- **PUVA and ultraviolet therapy.** Use of PUVA or ultraviolet treatments have helped some cases.
- **Capsaicin.** This cream may reduce the pain of aquagenic urticaria.
- **Stanozolol.** Some patients with HIV that have the symptoms of aquagenic urticaria have been helped with this medication.
- **Barrier methods.** Some have suggested bathing the skin with oil to protect it from exposure to water.

Those with this condition must constantly monitor what they eat and drink. They cannot drink water, tea, or coffee; colas appear to be the only thing they can tolerate. Certain fruits and vegetables with high water content are forbidden.

For Further Information

Gimenez-Arnau, Ana M., and Howard I. Maibach, eds. *Contact Urticaria Syndrome*. Boca Raton, FL: CRC Press, 2014.

Bell's Palsy: Partial Facial Paralysis

- Prevalence: Affects about 20 per 100,000 people
- Seldom hits before age 15 or after age 60
- Person experiences weakness or paralysis of facial muscles on one side of the face
- Condition usually only lasts about three weeks, then disappears on its own

Mike T. was riding his bike one pleasant February afternoon, and kept noting discomfort in his eyes. He thought it was dust from the dusty road, but when he got home later and looked in the mirror, he did not recognize himself. His face drooped, and the muscles on the left side of his face did not move. There were other annoying symptoms. Food fell out of the side of his mouth, and he could not pronounce words with the letters B, P, or F in them. His ear pained as sounds became louder. The doctor diagnosed him as having Bell's palsy, a condition he had never heard of. Then suddenly it went away, just as quickly as it had appeared.

WHAT IS BELL'S PALSY?

For some mysterious reason, the person experiences a weakness or paralysis of the facial muscles on one side of the face. The individual may feel that he or she has only half a face. It is usually temporary, and the exact cause has not been determined.

Bell's palsy results from the dysfunction or damage to one of the facial nerves. Two parts of the seventh cranial nerve run along through the fallopian canal on each side of the face. The fallopian canal is a long bony structure that travels through the face and controls muscle action of the face on one side. The nerve also controls eye opening and closing, blinking, smiling, and frowning. In Bell's palsy, messages that this nerve sends to the brain are disrupted, resulting in a variety of symptoms.

In 1829, Dr. Charles Bell (1774–1842), a Scottish physician and surgeon presented three cases to the Royal Society of London, in which he discussed the weakness and paralysis of one side of the face of some of his patients. As an anatomist, he traced it to one of the nerves that are located in the face. The condition was named for him, although the condition might have been described by earlier Greek, Roman, and Persian physicians. Other 19th-century physicians also described it.

Bell's palsy is one that continues to puzzle physicians. Several reasons for it have been proposed, none of them conclusive. The scientists generally agree that the facial nerve has been inflamed or damaged, but the exact causes are still unknown. Following are some of the proposed causes:

- Herpes simplex virus, the same one that causes fever blisters or cold sores
- Connections with certain illnesses such as flu, headaches, middle ear infections, diabetes, high blood pressure, sarcoidosis (a condition related to swelling of the lymph glands), or Lyme disease
- A latent virus related to varicella-zoster virus and Epstein-Barr virus. Both of these viruses are from the herpes family and are possibly triggered by environmental factors or emotional stress.
- Any trauma to the facial area

WHAT ARE THE SIGNS AND SYMPTOMS?

Many problems result when the facial nerve is involved. The first or main symptom is weakness or paralysis of the side of the face. It can be mild or severe. It is almost always on one side of the face, and rarely on both sides.

Other symptoms include a drooping eyelid, twitching of muscles of the face, drooping of the corner of the mouth, drooling, dryness of eye or mouth, excessive tearing in one eye, or impaired taste. Occasionally, in addition to pain around the mouth or jaw and behind the ear, the person may have headaches or extreme sensitivity to sound and dizziness. The person may have impaired speech and difficulty eating or drinking. In addition, the forehead muscles may be affected. Most of these symptoms begin suddenly and reach their peak within 48 hours to 72 hours.

HOW IS IT DIAGNOSED?

Many of the symptoms are similar to someone having a having a stroke. However, subtle differences do exist. Stroke will have other symptoms such as weakness, numbness, or tingling in the arms or legs. The person with Bell's palsy is unable to move the upper part of the forehead. A person with stroke can usually crinkle the forehead and move the upper part of the face.

Some of the symptoms may suggest Lyme disease, but this disease can be diagnosed by searching for Lyme-specific antibodies in the blood. Other conditions whose symptoms are similar include herpes zoster, sarcoidosis, and brain tumor.

If doctors can find an underlying condition for the palsy, then they will give it a name. However, if there is no reason, then it may be dubbed Bell's palsy. Bell's palsy appears to be a condition that is diagnosed by exclusion.

WHAT IS THE TREATMENT?

Most people regain normal face activity after about three weeks—even those who have gone without treatment. In a 1982 study when no treatment was available, Dr. E. Peitersen, a Danish neurosurgeon, followed 1,011 patients with Bell's palsy, and showed that 85 percent recovered after three weeks of onset. However, treatment and cases are individual. The treatments that have been most effective for more difficult cases are corticosteroids, such as prednisone. It appears to speed the recovery and should be begun within three days if possible. Using antivirals, such as acyclovir, does appear to be as effective, but only in about 7 percent of the cases; thus the possibility of the virus cause may still be viable.

For Further Information
Nemcoff, Marnie Suzanne. *Living with Bell's Palsy*. Reseda, CA: Glenneyre Press, 2011.

Bromhidrosis: Excessive Sweating and Body Odor

- Results in excessive sweating and body odor
- More prevalent in males
- May be more common in dark-skinned persons
- Probably has a genetic component

Joanne had great grades in high school, and was accepted sight unseen to nurse's training at the local community college. However, when she began to take classes, people sat on the other side of the room. She had no friends. When she would go into patients' rooms on clinical rounds, they would complain that her smell was making them sick. Although she was meticulous about grooming and had tried several deodorants, she still had the problem. Joanne had bromhidrosis, a condition that causes severe and permanent body odor.

WHAT IS BROMHIDROSIS?

Bromhidrosis is a medical condition that occurs when the skin gives off an abnormal and unpleasant, offensive smell, caused by the action of bacteria on the sweat. The condition can be personally and socially debilitating to the person, because the problem is often misunderstood, especially by those who do not have the condition. Like Joanne, the person may be avoided or may be the object of jokes about body odor.

So much misinformation exists. The person is considered dirty or may be accused of wearing unwashed clothes. With individuals with bromhidrosis, this is seldom the case. Even the origin of the word indicates unpleasantness. The word "bromhidrosis" comes from two Greek words: *bromos* meaning "the buck's stench" and *hidros* meaning "water" or "sweat."

Persons with bromhidrosis face discrimination in many ways. In 1994, the library at San Luis Obispo, California banned people with excessive body odor from their 14 branches. In another case, in 1989 Richard Kreimer of Morristown, New Jersey sued the public library because he was banned because of body odor. He won in federal court, but the appeals court reversed the decision, saying the patrons and staff should not have to endure the odor of another person. People with severe body odor cannot ride the bus in Honolulu, Hawaii; they face a $500 fine or six months in prison.

Bacteria working on perspiration produced by the sweat gland causes bromhidrosis. Sweat glands are divided into the following types:

- **Eccrine glands.** These glands are found over the entire body and are responsible for regulating body heat. In order to do so, they produce a normal, slightly salty, odorless secretion. When bacteria break down the perspiration, odor occurs. Also, other odors can come through the skin if certain substances such as garlic, curry, alcohol, or certain medications are taken.
- **Apocrine glands.** These glands are only in certain areas, such as the underarms, breasts, scalp, and groin area. The sweat is slightly oily and odorless at first, but within hours, bacteria that normally live on the skin break down the sweat, causing odor. The more bacteria that are present and the more perspiration that is produced, the greater the production of offensive body odor. Eccrine sweat softens the keratin in the skin, and when bacteria degrade this keratin/sweat combination, odor occurs. The major products of bacterial breakdown are fatty acids, such as butyric and formic acids, and ammonia. These compounds give the body a pungent odor. Apocrine bromhidrosis is the most common kind.

Several underlying causes have been identified. The person may have some metabolic dysfunction, such as renal or kidney failure. Genetics may play a part; certain bacterial skin flora may be passed down through families, along with hyperhidrosis, a condition of excess sweating. In addition, other causes such as obesity, diabetes, and certain rashes may contribute to the condition.

WHAT ARE THE SIGNS AND SYMPTOMS?

The main symptom is a bad body odor. Sometimes, but not always, it is present with hyperhidrosis, a condition in which the individual perspires profusely. Perspiration is produced by the sweat glands. When bacteria break down the perspiration, odor occurs. For those with bromhidrosis, the odor, which has been described as rancid, pungent, musty, or "sweet and sour," is extreme.

HOW IS IT DIAGNOSED?

The condition is obvious. The person has a distinct body odor and shows excessive sweating.

WHAT IS THE TREATMENT?

The treatment involves keeping the number of bacteria on the skin to a minimum and the skin as dry as possible. This may involve washing the armpits with a germicidal soap and removing hair from the area. Topical deodorants must be used, and clothing that "breathes" helps in the cooling process. Sometimes, the apocrine sweat glands may be removed by liposuction or by surgery. The person may require a special diet that includes abstinence from alcohol, nicotine, caffeine, and certain drugs.

For Further Information

Bartone, John C., ed. *Human Sweat and Sweating—Normal and Abnormal Including Hyperhidrosis and Bromhidrosis: Index of New Information and Guide-Book for Reference and Research.* Washington, DC: Abbe Pub Association of Washington, DC, 2001.

Burning Mouth Syndrome: A Mouth on Fire

- Also known as glossodynia; orodynia; oral dysaesthesia; glossopyrosis; stomatodynia
- Most prevalent in perimenopausal or postmenopausal women
- Reported in 10–40 percent of women seeking treatment for menopausal problems
- Burning sensation in the mouth, with no cause identified

Burning mouth syndrome (BMS) is a disorder characterized by burning or stinging of the tongue and mouth when the person has no other known disease. Its cause is basically unknown. People with certain other conditions may also have a burning mouth; this is known as secondary BMS.

WHAT IS BURNING MOUTH SYNDROME?

Burning mouth syndrome (BMS) is a very painful and frustrating condition that is described as a scalding, stinging, and/or itching sensation of the mouth and tongue. According to Netto, et al. in a 2011 study presented in *Clinical Oral Investigations*, it can last from four to six months, and involves mostly the tongue, with or without affecting the lips or the sides of the cheeks. Some people report it has lasted for years. Although it can affect both men and women, it is seen mostly in women who are going through menopause or who have finished their menstrual cycles. Some researchers correlate it with loss of the hormone estrogen, although this idea has not been completely validated.

Some doctors in the mid-19th century spoke about patients who described a condition in which the mouth and tongue felt like it was on fire, but it was not until a 1936 article in the *Journal of the American Medical Association* that it was given the name glossodynia, from the Greek words *gloss* meaning "tongue" and *dyn* meaning "pain." It has had several names since then, but was only recognized as a distinct disease by the International Headache Society in 2004.

BMS is classified as two types:

- **Primary.** This type is the idiopathic form, in which no organic cause can be identified; about 50 percent of the cases fall in this category. An idiopathic condition is one that arises spontaneously, for which there is no known cause.
- **Secondary.** A large number of disorders, including nutritional deficiencies and Parkinson's disease, may include symptoms of burning mouths.

No specific cause has been identified. However, there are a number of theories. The correlation with menopause and women suggests hormonal change as a cause. Other causes include: damage to nerves that control pain and taste, dry mouth from taking certain medications, nutritional deficiencies, allergies, oral candidiasis, which is a fungal infection of the mouth, acid reflux, poor-fitting dentures, and anxiety and depression. Some physicians consider it a psychosomatic illness, or that the person is a hypochondriac.

WHAT ARE THE SIGNS AND SYMPTOMS?

The pain is spontaneous and is described as burning, tingling, or scalding. It is generally ascribed to both sides of the tongue, palate, and lower lip and may be accompanied by a dry or sore mouth and a metallic taste. Likewise, three types of pain onset are described:

Type 1. In this type, symptoms are not present upon waking, but increase throughout the day.

Type 2. Symptoms are present when one awakes, and persist throughout the day.

Type 3. There is no regular pattern of symptoms.

Type two is the most common, with type three being the least common.
Because of the consistent and unpredictable pain symptoms, BMS is a debilitating disease that interferes with a person's quality of life.

HOW IS IT DIAGNOSED?

Before a making a diagnosis of primary BMS, physicians must rule out the possible secondary causes. If the condition is caused by something like an iron or vitamin deficiency, adding these nutrients to the diet may correct it. If it is caused by a fungal infection, this can be treated. Thus, primary BMS is a disease of exclusion.

WHAT IS THE TREATMENT?

The first order is to identify whether there is another existing disorder, such as diabetes, Sjögren's syndrome, or a thyroid problem, and treat those conditions. With successful treatment of many of these disorders, the mouth burning may subside.

If no correlation with another disorder is made, the main treatment is to alleviate the symptoms. Medications such as benzodiazepine, tricyclic antidepressant, gabapentin, and topical capsaicin have helped.

The website from the National Institutes of Health suggests some self-help tips to relieve the burning pain:

- Sip water frequently
- Suck on ice cubes
- Avoid hot spicy foods and products that are high in acid, such as citrus fruits and juices
- Avoid mouthwashes that contain alcohol
- Chew sugarless gum
- Brush teeth and dentures with baking soda and water
- Avoid alcohol and tobacco products

For Further Information

Scala, A., L. Checchi, M. Montevecchi, I. Marini, and M. A. Giamberardino. 2003. "Update on Burning Mouth Syndrome: Overview and Patient Management." *Critical Review of Oral Biology and Medicine* 14: 275–91.

Charles Bonnet Syndrome: I Can't See, But I Do See

- Also known as phantom eye syndrome
- People who have lost sight vividly see things that are not there
- Those affected are not mentally ill
- Hallucinations have a physical explanation

Charles Bonnet (1720–1793) was a philosopher who resided in Switzerland. He cared for his visually impaired 87-year-old grandfather, who reported seeing things. Bonnet knew that his grandfather was mentally stable and completely alert. When he described pictures of men, women, birds, or buildings, he knew that the hallucinations were the result of his grandfather not being able to see. Bonnet wrote an essay about the condition in French in 1760. His writings about the disorder were not found until the 1980s, when Charles Bonnet syndrome (CBS) was recognized as a distinct disorder.

Bonnet was the first to make the connection between vision loss and the visual hallucinations; the condition was named for him.

WHAT IS CHARLES BONNET SYNDROME?

Charles Bonnet syndrome is a phenomenon of those who have once been able to see, but have lost their sight through some occurrence. They are not mentally ill, and do not have dementia or other disorders that may cause the hallucinations. They report seeing very vivid items, such as geometric shapes, swirling colors, animals, plants, changes in the landscape, and people who are usually smaller than in real life. People have even described buses driving into the living room and people sitting on the couch beside them. According to a study done by Dr. Oliver Sacks, author of the book *Hallucinations*, the most common images are of faces or cartoons. These pictures are very vivid and appear in much more detail than the person could ever remember seeing when he or she had sight. The person understands that these are hallucinations, and are not real.

A hallucination is different from a delusion, which originates in the mind. A hallucination relates only to the senses. The sense related to Charles Bonnet syndrome is only sight, and does not appear with the other senses, such as hearing, taste, smell, or touch.

Blindness can be caused by several types of conditions: cataracts, glaucoma, macular degeneration, diabetes, and eye injuries. If a person is isolated or extremely sensory deprived, CBS may be more likely. Other things that can worsen the visual hallucinations are stroke, depression, and grief. The following specific cause is only a theory: although there is a true lack of visual input into the brain, the brain still releases images. This phenomenon is possibly similar to the phantom limb syndrome, in which a person may feel his or her leg, even though the limb is amputated. This theory comes from a study of 13 sighted people who were blindfolded for five days and deprived of visual stimulation. L. B. Merabet, et al. in the *Journal of Psychopathology* found that of these patients, 10 reported hallucinations after the first day.

WHAT ARE THE SIGNS AND SYMPTOMS?

The underlying symptom is the loss of vision, with the primary symptom being visual hallucinations. These visions are very different from those with psychiatric disorders, in that the pictures are quite pleasant and very vivid. People with mental disorders appear to have more disturbing hallucinations.

HOW IS IT DIAGNOSED?

Many of the people with this condition are misdiagnosed, because the people are embarrassed to talk about hallucination, believing that people will consider them crazy or that they are not being truthful. The story that is told in the sidebar describes how a doctor who had read about CBS in a medical journal diagnosed it properly.

WHAT IS THE TREATMENT?

There is no test for CBS; however, the nature of the hallucination should be a clue. The diagnosis usually occurs in older people with damage to the eye structure or to optic pathways. One of the common conditions is macular degeneration, a condition in which the central focus of the eye is lost but peripheral vision may be maintained. An eye physician should be consulted for the proper treatment of the eye condition. Drugs to treat certain conditions may also evoke the hallucinations; therefore, a close look at medications should be taken. Many people do not want to tell anyone about the hallucinations, because they are embarrassed and afraid that others will think they have some type of mental illness.

Likewise, there is no specific treatment for CBS. If the person is judged to be of sound mind and a clear thinker, it is important to emphasize that this is an happening to people who are visually impaired.

CASE HISTORY: ROSEMARY M. ENCOURAGES KNOWLEDGE ABOUT CBS

Many doctors are completely unaware of Charles Bonnet syndrome (CBS), and therefore do not help patients who describe seeing things that are not there.

Rosemary, a 92-year-old resident of Gainesville, Florida, lost her sight from macular degeneration of the eyes. When she told her doctor about the hallucinations she was having, no one knew what to tell her. However, one of her attending physicians was a young resident in ophthalmology. When he heard her description of the things that she saw, he remembered reading about a condition called Charles Bonnet syndrome. The resident realized that Rosemary was stable and lucid and did not have dementia. She fit the description of CBS perfectly.

What a relief it was for Rosemary to put a name on the disorder. It was a real weight off her shoulders to realize that the hallucinations were not dangerous, and were common in people with low vision.

Now her mission is telling people with low vision about Charles Bonnet syndrome, so they do not "fear the worse" and have to keep silent. She also informs the doctors she meets that she has had CBS. She has found that primary care and "younger doctors" are more responsive than eye specialists and older doctors.

Rosemary gives this advice: If you think you may have CBS, go to your doctor's appointment armed with one or two articles that explain what you are experiencing. Let them know, so they can help others understand what is happening to them.

For Further Information

Vukicevic M., and K. Fitzmaurice. 2008. "Butterflies and Black Lacy Patterns: The Prevalence and Characteristics of Charles Bonnet Hallucinations in an Australian Population." *Clinical and Experimental Ophthalmology* 36: 659–65.

Foreign Accent Syndrome: Sounds Different to Me

- Person begins speaking with a foreign accent
- Usually the result of a stroke, but can be caused by other types of head trauma
- Since 1947, 30 cases reported in medical literature worldwide
- No known treatment

What if you were to wake up one day and start talking as if you were a Russian, German, or Swede? That is what happened to Cindy Lou Romberg, a Washington State native, who fell out of a moving truck in 1981. She rolled her R's like a Russian, chopped syllables like a German, and could not pronounce a W, just like a Swede. She has never been out of her native Washington. Yet, she has foreign accent syndrome, a condition that people know little about.

WHAT IS FOREIGN ACCENT SYNDROME?

Foreign accent syndrome (FAS) is a rare medical condition in which people pronounce words with a foreign accent. It is usually the result of a head trauma, stroke, migraines, or some other developmental problem. When the person regains consciousness from the event, their speech sounds different and foreign. The person does not actually acquire fluency in that language, although there have been claims to the contrary. Several instances of FAS have been reported in the news media, and are always of great interest.

The French neurologist Pierre Marie (1853–1940) first described the condition in 1909. The first confirmed case of foreign accent syndrome occurred in August 1917, when a 16-year-old Kentucky girl awoke after a coma and began speaking with a strong English accent. The family and friends thought that she was afflicted with a "devil's disease" and should be punished. Her parents contacted Georg Monrad-Krohn (1850–1931), a Norwegian neurologist who agreed to cure her of her accent. When he had no success, he gave up and suggested that they accept their daughter as she was. However, Monrad-Krohn became interested in the condition, and his research contributed to the development of the new field of neurolinguistics.

FAS is not listed in any edition of the *Diagnostic and Statistical Manual of Mental Disorders*, and is only briefly mentioned in textbooks for those studying speech pathology. It is not a condition that is considered mental or psychological in nature.

FAS may be the result of several happenings: stroke, traumatic brain injury, multiple lesions, epilepsy, migraines, and multiple sclerosis. Also, the origin may not be known. FAS after stroke may be related to a network of brain processes associated with speech production.

The brain consists of two halves, called hemispheres. A pertinent analogy is the walnut. It has two sides or halves that look somewhat alike, but not exactly. In most individuals, the left side of the brain is the center of language abilities. Damage to this area can cause speech problems. One area, called Broca's area, is located in the left hemisphere towards the back and bottom of the frontal lobe. A condition known as aphasia occurs when the person cannot express himself in speech. Broca's aphasia is a nonfluent type, associated with the inability to make certain sounds, called apraxia. A person with apraxia has difficulty speaking, because the tongue, vocal cords, jaw, and lips do not form the correct patterns to produce words. FAS speech may resemble that of other disorders, but they do not sound like that to the listener. Instead, people just perceive it as a foreign accent.

Other researchers think that the problem may arise in the cerebellum, the part of the brain located at the back of the brain that controls motor function. This idea supports the notion that the problem patterns are mechanical and nonspecific.

WHAT ARE THE SIGNS AND SYMPTOMS?

The person wakes up from the accident or coma speaking with a foreign accent. To one who is untrained, the accent definitely appears that way; however, those who are linguists have a different outlook. Experts understand that the change in the way the person is speaking is due to a change within a part of the brain that alters pitch or intonation. Other symptoms may include changes in the individual's personality, within 34 to 48 hours after waking up. The way the person spoke previously may disappear within 72 hours, with the transformation to the new accent made within four days.

In 1941, German bombs were falling over Oslo, Norway. A large piece of shrapnel flew into the head of Astrid L., a 30-year-old civilian. She was in a coma for several days, and when she recovered, she had a strong German accent, something that was not too popular at the time. In fact, she was shunned by her fellow countrymen. However, her case became a landmark. The injury she sustained was on the right side of the brain, leading researchers to gather information about the condition and to realize that this was a medical condition. Monrad-Krohn reported the case history in a medical journal in 1947 and referred to it as foreign accent syndrome. Since this landmark case, over 40 instances have been described. Some accent changes that are documented are from Japanese to Korean, British to French, American English to British, and Spanish to Hungarian. The people do not sound abnormal to the listener, and it appears only that they have a foreign accent.

HOW IS IT DIAGNOSED?

The area of speech pathology is quite complex. Several specialists, including speech-language experts, neurologists, neuropsychologists, and psychologists may be involved. Many tests are given, including images of the brain with MRI (magnetic resonance imaging), CT (computed tomography), SPECT (single-photon emission computed tomography), or PET (positron emission tomography) scans. An EEG (electroencephalogram) may be used to measure the activity of the brain waves.

WHAT IS THE TREATMENT?

Because there are so few cases, few people are studying the condition. One place that is involved is the Callier Center for Communication Disorders at the University of Texas, Dallas. A team of researchers there believe that studying FAS will give clues to understanding speech difficulties in general.

For Further Information

Ryalls, Jack, and Nick Miller. *Foreign Accent Syndromes: The Stories People Have to Tell.* London: Psychology Press, 2015.

Guillain-Barre Syndrome: Ascending Paralysis

- Rare, only one or two cases per 100,000 people annually
- A neurological disorder in which the body's immune system attacks the peripheral nervous system
- Can strike people of any age and either sex
- No cure, but several treatment strategies are available

In 1976, the swine flu was making its way through the nation, and many people were vaccinated to protect against this outbreak. During the outbreak, and a few weeks after vaccination, some individuals began to feel very ill, with muscle weakness and tingling in the legs and feet that began in the lower extremities, then started ascending through the body. Researchers suspected that these symptoms might be related to the vaccine. The presentation of the disease and its symptoms was rare, and doctors in the emergency rooms had not seen cases with these exact symptoms. The name Guillain-Barre syndrome emerged. Although there was lots of concern at the time, the Centers for Disease Control and Prevention (CDC) noted that after studies of cases and epidemiology, the overall increase of cases was only 1 per 100,000 over the normal caseload.

WHAT IS GUILLAIN-BARRE SYNDROME?

Guillain-Barre syndrome (GBS) is an autoimmune disease in which the person's own body attacks part of the peripheral nervous system. This attack leads to inflammation that causes muscle weakness and tingling in the legs, the first symptoms of GBS. GBS can occur at any age; however, the risk tends to increase with every decade of age by 20 percent.

In 1916, Georges Guillain (1876–1961), Alexander Barre (1880–1967), and André Strohl (1887–1977) researched a disease that was found in two French soldiers in World War I. The three carefully recorded and interpreted the muscle reflexes of the patients, and found it was associated with the peripheral nervous system. Spinal taps revealed an increase of spinal proteins, but the cell count was normal. The first detailed study was published in 1916, but Strohl's contributions were not acknowledged. In 1927, only Gillian and Barre published the final paper of their findings. Although the French physician Jean Baptiste Octave Landry (1828–1865) first described the disorder in 1859, the condition was named for Guillain and Barre. Although GBS is a rare disorder, it does show up from time to time; it was never proven to be related to the swine flu vaccine.

Actually, no one knows the cause. They do know it is not contagious. Why the immune system begins to attack itself is a mystery. In normal circumstances, the immune system is a friend guarding against unwelcome invaders. But in GBS, the immune bodies begin to destroy the myelin sheath that surrounds the axons of the nerve bodies. The cells of the nervous system are made of a cell body, dendrites, which receive the impulses, and axons, threadlike fibers that carry the nerve signals. The axons are covered with a slick white sheath, which speeds up the transition of the nerve signals over long distances. If something interrupts myelin, the signals do not get to their destination in the muscles, and weakness and tingling occur. That is what happens when the myelin sheath is attacked by antibodies from the immune system.

Two-thirds of the people with GBS have some type of infection before the onset. Most common are gastrointestinal disorders and respiratory infections. Some cases have been suspected to have been triggered by influenza vaccines. There was a connection in a 1976 outbreak of swine flu, in which the vaccine appears to have been incriminated. However, since then there have been few suspected cases related to vaccines.

WHAT ARE THE SIGNS AND SYMPTOMS?

GBS may develop rapidly and worsen quickly. In a few cases, it may take several days to develop. The primary symptom is loss of muscle function or paralysis in the legs and feet, which then progresses to the arms. It can then progress to other parts of the body. This is why it is called ascending paralysis, because eventually the body is paralyzed. When the body trunk is paralyzed, it is life-threatening, because respiration is affected and low blood pressure may accompany abnormal heart rate. The person will lose tendon reflexes in the arms and legs, and have muscle tenderness or pain with uncoordinated movements. Other symptoms may include blurred vision, palpitations, and difficulty moving facial muscles.

HOW IS IT DIAGNOSED?

Although several disorders may have the same symptoms as GBS, it is essential that this condition be diagnosed in reasonable time. If the person reports being very ill, along with muscle weakness and tingling legs, GBS should be suspected. In addition to low blood pressure and heart rate, the reflexes of ankle and knee jerk reaction do not respond. Tests may include the following: a spinal tap, an electrocardiogram to check activity of the heart, an electromyography to test electrical activity in muscles, a nerve conduction velocity test, and pulmonary function tests.

WHAT IS THE TREATMENT?

There is no cure. However, there are several strategies for treatment. When the disorder is suspected, a plasma exchange called electrophoresis and high-dose immunoglobulin therapy are used. In electrophoresis, the entire blood is removed and processed so that red and white blood cells are separated from the plasma, where the questionable antibodies may be found. The blood cells are then put back in the body, which will replace the lost plasma. Scientists are not sure why immunoglobulin therapy appears to work so well.

Other treatments may be used. Breathing support and a ventilator may be necessary. Blood thinners may prevent clots, and pain medication may help problems in these areas. Physical therapy is necessary to help joints and muscles remain healthy. Recovery may take quite a while, and there can always be complications.

For Further Information

Langton, Brian S. *A First Step: Understanding Guillain-Barre Syndrome.* New York: Trafford Publishing, 2006.

Laryngopharyngeal Reflux (LRP): Silent Reflux

- Prevalence: Overlooked and misdiagnosed; affects over 50 million Americans
- Occurs when gastric juices back up and pool in the back of the throat
- Different from gastroesophageal reflux disease or GERD
- Person may not have heartburn as they do with GERD

Mary Ann is a 55-year-old school guidance counselor. She began to notice that every morning, she woke up with a very coarse throat that persisted through the day. By the end of the day, her voice was very tired and raspy, but she though it was because she talked to people all day. She never had heartburn. When she went to the Mayo Clinic, the doctors informed her that she had silent reflux, a disorder that is usually missed in diagnosis; however, it is quite common.

WHAT IS LARYNGOPHARYNGEAL REFLUX?

The stomach is the main organ where digestion of proteins begins to take place. The stomach has a weak form of hydrochloric acid (HCl) and pepsin, a gastric juice. A favorite experiment in high school biology is to take a little piece of meat and suspend it in a test tube with the HCl and pepsin. When the student looks at the result the next day, the meat is almost completely dissolved. This is what happens to begin the breakdown of the protein food that you eat. The acid is kept in the stomach by a muscle called the lower esophageal sphincter (LES) muscle.

Gastroesophageal reflux (GERD) was first recognized in the mid-1930s, and is now the most prevalent of all gastrointestinal (GI) disorders. However it was not until 1968 that J. Cherry reported acid-related lesions in the larynx. The condition was then referred to as the Cherry-Donner syndrome. In 1979 Pellegrini and DeMeester linked the larynx condition and hoarseness to reflux.

When the LES muscle does not work properly, acid and stomach juices will wash back into the esophagus and even into the throat and voice box. The term "reflux" comes from a Greek word meaning "back flow." GERD is a commonly known condition that occurs when the juices back into the esophagus. The skin on the esophagus is just like the back of your hand, and is very easily burned by the acid. This burning sensation is called heartburn, although it has nothing to do with the heart. If the juices move quickly though the esophagus, they may land in the throat and pool in the back of the throat in an area called the pharynx and larynx or voice box.

Thus, the term laryngopharyngeal reflux (LPR) refers to the condition when the stomach contents slip through the LES, move quickly through the esophagus, and then locates in the throat. Compared to the esophagus, which is sensitive like the skin on the back of the hand, the folds of the voice box and surrounding tissues are even more sensitive. The person may not even know that it exists, except for the hoarse throat.

WHAT ARE THE SIGNS AND SYMPTOMS?

Several symptoms may be present, or just one or two of the symptoms. The person notices hoarseness that never seems to go away. He or she may have a dry cough, trouble swallowing, too much throat mucus, or a lump in the throat that feels like something is stuck in the throat. Some people may completely lose their voice. Others may have postnasal drip, a feeling that there is always some mucus gathering in the back of the throat. Some people with LPR may find swallowing difficult, have indigestion, wheezing, or a chronic cough that wakes them from sleep.

Other symptoms may also be present. Some adults have an acid taste in their throats, especially on awaking, or the throat may have a burning sensation. Also, some patients may have sinus trouble and difficulty breathing. The list also includes difficulty swallowing, shortness of breath, snoring, sleep apnea, bad breath, tooth decay, asthma, and COPD. Throat cancer can occur if untreated for a prolonged time.

HOW IS IT DIAGNOSED?

Unfortunately, many doctors do not recognize the symptoms of this disease, and that the patient should be treated by a trained reflux specialist in a new medical specialty called integrated aerodigestive medicine. Doctors in this area believe that LPR is a silent epidemic.

Sometimes the condition mimics asthma. A simple test can note the difference. People with reflux have trouble getting air in when they breathe in; people with asthma have trouble getting air out. If the condition is misdiagnosed, medication for asthma will not help.

The symptoms alone are not reliable to diagnose the condition. After a detailed history and examination of the throat area, the doctor will use an instrument called a flexible fiberoptic laryngoscope to look at the throat and larynx. The person with LPR will have very inflamed and red vocal folds. If symptoms are severe, the doctor may use a test called an ambulatory 24-hour pH monitoring device, which is a small tube inserted through the nose into the esophagus. This tube collects and measures the amount of acid through a tube connected to a small computer within a 24-hour period.

WHAT IS THE TREATMENT?

Management of the symptoms is sometimes difficult, but is curable. When there is a definite diagnosis, certain behavioral changes involving weight loss and dietary changes may help. Following are the four general treatments:

- **Posture changes and weight reduction.**

- **Healthy eating.** First, no late night eating and no overeating; going to bed with a full stomach pushes the acid back up into the esophagus. The person should not eat at least three hours before going to bed. Second, restrict all acidic foods, such as citrus fruits and drinks. Soft or carbonated drinks have a weak acid called carbonic acid. Do not drink anything out of a bottle except water. The diet should be both low fat and low acid. Foods such as mints, chocolate, tomato-based products, red wine, caffeine, and fried foods add to reflux. No smoking or alcohol. Reading the labels is essential. Signs that foods may be acidic include anything that adds phosphoric acid, ascorbic acid, citric acid or "vitamin C enhanced."
- **Medications that reduce stomach acid.** The most common prescriptions are proton pump inhibitors such as AcipHex, Nexium, Prevacid, Prilosec, or Zegerid. Other are called H2 blockers; these include Axid, Pepcid, Tagamet, and Zantac. Antacids, such as Tums or Rolaids, may help neutralize acid.
- **Surgery to prevent reflux.** This is generally rare, but necessary for some extreme cases. Called fundoplication, this surgery wraps the upper part of the stomach around the lower esophagus to create a stronger valve between the stomach, which will control stomach acids. Another surgical procedure involves placing a ring of titanium beads around the outside of the lower esophagus. This strengthens the valve, but still lets food pass through.

PREVENTING REFLUX

- Smoking can cause reflux. Do not smoke.
- Avoid wearing any constricting clothing or a band around the waist.
- Do not eat at a late hour. Plan to have your last meal at least three hours before going to bed.
- Practice portion control. Do not eat large meals.
- Lose weight. Pressure of excess fat, particularly belly fat, puts excess pressure on the area of the lower esophageal sphincter (LES).
- Know what foods to avoid. Following are a partial list: caffeine, carbonated beverages, citrus and citrus drinks, tomato-based foods, mints, alcohol of any types, cheese, fried foods, eggs, chocolate.
- If sleeping is affected or symptoms or more severe, elevate the head of the bed about six inches.
- Chewing gum may increase production of saliva and neutralize acid.

For Further Information

Zerbib, F., and D. Stoll. 2010. "Management of Laryngopharyngeal Reflux: An Unmet Medical Need." *Neurogastroenterol Motil* 22 (2): 109–12.

Moebius Syndrome: A Person with a Mask-like Face

- Rare congenital condition in which the face is paralyzed
- Prevalence: 2 to 20 cases per million births; about 2,000 cases worldwide
- Related to underdevelopment of cranial nerves VI and VII
- No specific treatment

A story that has as its heroine a person with a paralyzed face could only be a fanciful tale of magic and intrigue. That is the plot of Eliza Wyatt's novella *Painted*. The author weaves an imaginative story about a girl who has an unusual appearance, in that she has no facial movements. Wyrren Jadis, an heir to a duchy of her country, has been banned from her fictional country and is living on the charity of the ruler of Hael Malstrom. When someone threatens to kill the king, she is determined to find out why, and is involved in the solution to a magical mystery. The protagonist heroine has Moebius syndrome.

WHAT IS MOEBIUS SYNDROME?

Moebius syndrome is a congenital condition in which the person is born with no facial expression or eye movements. This nonprogressive condition results from the underdevelopment of certain nerves. Cranial nerves merge directly from the brain and brainstem. The nerves are assigned Roman numerals I–XII, and control various functions from the sensory organs and glands or internal organs. In Moebius syndrome, cranial nerves VI and VII are underdeveloped. These are the nerves that control eye movement and facial expression. Sometimes other nerves such as III, IV, V, IX, X, and XII may be involved. If VIII is affected, hearing loss will also occur.

Most children with this disorder are not able to close their eyes or create any facial expression. In addition, they may have limb or chest wall abnormalities. The children generally have normal intelligence, but because of their lack of expression may be considered less able or intelligent.

Paul Julius Moebius (1853–1907) was a German neurologist from Leipzig who was a prolific writer and student in the field of neurophysiology and endocrinology. He published the first study of children who had mask-like faces in 1888. The syndrome was named for him. The children with the mask-like faces may have other physical problems.

However, several theories as to the cause of the underdevelopment have been debated. Moebius theorized that there was degenerative or toxic damage to the cranial nerve. The damage was the result of the loss of blood flow during prenatal development. That loss of blood affected the cranial nerves as they were developing. Some scientists speculate that there is a genetic component; the disorder appears to be connected with changes in regions of chromosome 3, 10, or 13.

Some noxious event during pregnancy may cause the disorder. Use of cocaine by the mother is believed to have vascular effects of causing the loss of blood flow during fetal formation. Some doctors speculate that misoprostol, a widely used drug used to induce abortions in Brazil, Argentina, and sometimes in the United States, may cause Moebius. Although the procedure is successful in 90 percent of cases, the drug could affect some of the 10 percent in which it is not effective.

WHAT ARE THE SIGNS AND SYMPTOMS?

The symptoms depend on what cranial nerves are affected, but VI and VII are damaged in all cases. If other cranial nerves are involved, other symptoms may appear.

The condition will be obvious at birth or in the first few weeks or months. The child lacks facial expression and will have difficulty sucking and feeding. He or she may not be able to follow objects with the eyes, but instead may move the entire head to follow the object. He cannot move his eyes laterally. In addition, the eyelids may not close completely so that it appears that she is sleeping with her eyes open. He will not be able to blink. Because of the paralysis of facial muscles, the child may drool, and may throw her head back in order to swallow. This can be a real problem, because the child may take bits of food or drink into the lungs, causing a condition known as aspirational pneumonia. This can lead to death at an early age.

Certain other problems may be noted early. The child may have limb abnormalities, such as clubbed feet or missing fingers or toes, crossed-eyes, and chest-wall abnormalities. Because of the difficulty in blinking, the cornea of the eye may be chronically irritated.

The children may also have serious dental problems. A small mouth may result in crowding of teeth as they begin to come in, and dental surgery must be performed. These surgeries are usually done after the ages of 12 to 14 years. Also, after this, they may have so-called smile surgery, in which muscles from the thigh are transferred to the corners of the mouth, helping the child to smile.

HOW IS IT DIAGNOSED?

Although Moebius syndrome is rare and has specific symptoms, it is often misdiagnosed or undiagnosed. Parents usually note the first symptoms, and note the mask-like appearance, and that the child cannot smile. However, there are a number of other conditions that it may be confused with, including birth trauma, Kallmann syndrome, or metabolic neuropathy. No laboratory tests help with this diagnosis. Many of the children are diagnosed with autism, and although it is true that about

10–20 percent of children with Moebius may have autism, the misdiagnosis may keep children from being treated for other symptoms.

WHAT IS THE TREATMENT?

Because there is no single course of treatment, supportive measures must be used to treat the various symptoms. For example, if feeding problems exist, there are special bottles to help. Physical, speech, and occupational therapy may help. Dental attention is essential. The smile surgery can affect the ability to smile, but this 12-hour procedure only helps the appearance of the mouth, and does not affect the rest of the facial muscles.

For Further Information

Phillips, Kiowana E. *The Boy Who Smiles with His Heart (A Moebius Syndrome Story)*. Raleigh, NC: Lulu.com, 2014.

Morgellons: Disease or Delusion?

- Itchy burning skin, with threadlike fibers appearing on the skin
- Thousands of people have reported symptoms in 50 states and other countries
- Medical community doubts it exists
- No standardized treatment

People with Morgellons (pronounced with a hard "g") describe a condition in which the skin feels like it is burning, itching, or crawling, along with appearance of thread-like fibers that appear under the skin. Thousands of people have reported the condition in all 50 states and throughout the world, including Europe, Japan, South Africa, and the Philippines. The only problem is that the medical community cannot find any evidence for the condition and doubts that it exists.

WHAT IS MORGELLONS?

Morgellons is the name given to describe this condition characterized first by crawling sensations under the skin, then by sores that have fibers or threads that emerge. The condition appears more often in Caucasian women between the ages of 35 and 40.

Before 2002, no one had ever heard of this condition. Mary Leitao, a biologist from McMurray, Pennsylvania, noted these unusual symptoms that plagued both her and her son. She began to research and found a 17th-century medical text in which Sir Thomas Browne (1604–1682) wrote in "A Letter to a Friend" in 1690, telling about several medical conditions affecting the skin in children in Languedoc, France. He called this condition "endemial distemper." The children broke out with coarse hairs on their backs called "the Morgellons." Later, in 1935, C. E. Kellett (1908–1978), a British doctor, connected Morgellons with a French term *mascious*, meaning "little flies." The exact connection with these two terms and the occurrences today is not clear. Leitao chose this name and uses it to refer to the condition when she addresses physicians and politicians.

So many unknown factors surround Morgellons. It is not recognized as a clinical disease. So why does a person get this disorder, if it is a disorder. Some patients have connected it with Lyme disease (see Case History). Some health care practitioners have called it "unexplained dermopathy," meaning there is no explanation for the condition. Others believe it is all in the mind of the person, and connect it with a condition called "delusional parasitosis," in which people mistakenly believe they have insects crawling under their skin.

WHAT ARE THE SIGNS AND SYMPTOMS?

Morgellons is not listed as a disease, and physicians currently do not have specific criteria for diagnosis. People usually diagnose the condition themselves and gather information about it from the internet. In fact, someday this may be considered one of the first diseases created and spread by the internet.

Following are the symptoms that a person with Morgellons may describe:

- Bugs are crawling all over the skin.
- The skin is burning and stinging, with intense itching.
- Black, stringy fibers may be embedded in the skin or may project out of the skin.
- Sores may appear that heal very slowly.
- The person is very tired and has difficulty paying attention,
- He or she may have other physical symptoms, such as muscle or joint pain, hair loss, nervous disorders, or memory loss.

Because of the intense itching and other symptoms, individuals have a poor quality of life.

HOW IS IT DIAGNOSED?

Dr. Rhonda Casey, chief of pediatrics at Oklahoma State University Medical Center, was one of the first to call for an investigation of Morgellons. Responding to the concern of the medical profession, the U.S. Centers for Disease Control and

Prevention (CDC) released a study on January 25, 2002. The study published in the journal *PLOS One* screened 115 patients from Northern California and found the following:

- The items in the skin are not alive; they are not insects or mites.
- The fibers are pieces of cotton or cellulose from clothing or bandages.
- Roughly 40 percent of the skin samples showed chronic irritation, probably from scratching.
- Drugs were detected in hair samples from half of the patients.
- About one-third had some type of neuropsychiatric condition.

INTERVIEW WITH "CHERIE," ALBANY, NEW YORK

Cherie (who wishes only to be identified by her first name) is a hospital executive living in Albany, New York. In an interview, she tells how she is convinced that Morgellons disease is real, and relates her struggle with the medical profession that she is a part of:

It was February 2012, and I was on a cruise. I looked in the mirror to check out the itching sensation on my neck. What an unusual sight. What I saw were the tips of little pointy red and blue things sticking out of the skin on my neck and in the crown of my head. When I got back from the cruise, I started swabbing the skin, but the tiny fluorescent fibers were everywhere. I had never seen or heard anything like this in my 52 years. I called my husband to look and he agreed—they were there—everywhere.

When I started talking to people at the hospital, they thought I was crazy, and gave me all the medical talk about parasites and imagination. They totally denied that this was a condition. I even took a sample to my dermatologist, who said it was delusional parasitosis. He said that I had worn a red sweater, and these are the fibers.

During the month of March, things started advancing. The fibers crept and melted into my skin, forming a gel-like lesion that sometimes bled. What is worse, my son, who was 14 at the time, had fibers coming out of pores of his skin.

I turned to the internet to see what I could find. After much research, I found a site for Dr. Virginia Savely, a [doctorate] nurse practitioner (DNP) from Texas who now lives in Washington, DC. She is one of the leading professionals who is treating Lyme disease and the new Morgellons disease. Dr. Savely believes there is a connection between latent Lyme disease and Morgellons.

I went to see her in June. She verified the thousands of tiny blue and red fibers on the neck. After running some tests, I did test positive for past Lyme infection, which were not active but latent. Yes, my son and I had both had tick bites, and we remembered ticks and a wasp bite with a bull's eye, one of the signs of Lyme disease. I was given high dose antibiotics and antifungals to attack the biofilm, the gel-like lesions on my skin. Insurance pays for none of this; I have spent thousands of dollars.

I do believe that the disfiguring of my skin and some cognitive decline is due to Morgellons. There are thousands out there just like me. So I will continue to be an advocate and believe there is an answer out there.

The study ruled out the possibility of insects, infections, or environmental causes. However, they did indicate additional studies into nerve damage or other causes were in order.

WHAT IS THE TREATMENT?

Although there is no specific diagnosis and consequently no cure, treating the symptoms has been beneficial. Some medications that treat tics or psychosis such as olanzapine or pimozide may help. A variety of anti-itch medications may also be used for relief.

For Further Information
Devine, Bobbi. *Morgellons Among Us.* Bloomington, IN: Xlibris, 2014.

Multiple System Atrophy: When All Systems Fail

- Also known as Shy-Drager syndrome, and neurogenic orthostatic hypotension
- Rare condition affecting 15,000 to 50,000 Americans
- Similar to Parkinson's, but inflicts more widespread damage to organ systems
- There is no cure

Living in a Florida retirement community, Grace was extremely pleased to be away from the ice and snow of New England. However, she began to note that she had a combination of symptoms that included slow and erratic movements and problems with heart and breathing. At first the doctors thought she had Parkinson's disease, but were puzzled by the other systems that were involved. They then proclaimed she had a rare disease called multiple system atrophy. This disease is little known, and underdiagnosed.

WHAT IS MULTIPLE SYSTEM ATROPHY?

Multiple system atrophy (MSA) is a progressive neurological disorder that affects the autonomic nervous system, which controls involuntary actions and movement. Sometimes the condition is referred to as Parkinson-Plus syndrome, which means the symptoms of Parkinson's are there, but other systems are also affected. Also, it is distinguished from Parkinson's, in that the person does not respond to the dopamine medications, a staple in treating that disease.

The cause is unknown, and the vast number of cases are sporadic, meaning they occur at random. There is one distinguishing feature that is present in many of the cases. A protein called alpha-synuclein accumulates in the glia, the cells that support the nerve cells in the brain. Occurring in the area that makes the myelin sheath of the nerve cells, α-synuclein can affect the coating of the nerve cells that enables them to conduct electrical messages. A-synuclein is also present in Parkinson's, but is found within the nerve cells and not in the glia that support them. The location of α-synuclein may account for the difference in symptoms. There is also a theory advanced that variations in the gene *SCNA* may be responsible for the differences.

WHAT ARE THE SIGNS AND SYMPTOMS?

MSA damages the nervous system. First, the person begins to move slowly, and has tremors and stiffness. These symptoms are similar to the beginning stages of Parkinson's disease. Then, the person notices that he is clumsy and uncoordinated. Others may notice that she has a croaky or quivering voice. There are problems with bladder control, when the person has the sudden urge to urinate but has difficulty emptying the bladder. Many other problems could occur, such as nausea and digestive problems, sleep-related difficulties, and confusion or dementia.

Symptoms that tend to appear when the person is in their fifties advance rapidly over a five to 10 year period. MSA tends to progress more rapidly than Parkinson's, and most people require some assistive aides for walking only a few years after the diagnosis is made. The person usually dies of heart failure or pneumonia, because of lung or breathing issues.

Researchers divide the symptoms into two types:

- **MSA-P or the Parkinson's type.** This type progresses similar to Parkinson's; the individual moves slowly, with stiffness and tremors. Added are other neurological problems, such as those affecting balance, coordination, and autonomic nervous system dysfunction.
- **MSA-C or the cerebellar type.** The cerebellum is an area at the back of the brain that controls the automatic processes. With this type, the person has problems with balance and coordination, difficulty swallowing, speech abnormalities, and abnormal eye movements.

Some other obvious symptoms may also occur. Contractures are conditions that occur when the muscles and tendons around the joints shorten, and the person cannot move the hands or limbs easily. An abnormal posture called the Pisa syndrome can occur, in which the body leans to one side, like the leaning Tower of Pisa. The person may develop antecolis, a condition in which the neck bends forward and the head drops down. The individual may also have involuntary sighing or gasping.

HOW IS IT DIAGNOSED?

The diagnosis is quite difficult and at first may be confused with Parkinson's. The physicians will take a history, perform a battery of autonomic testing, including blood pressure and heart rate, bladder function, and neuroimaging with MRI (magnetic resonance imaging) or PET (positron emission tomography) scan. The PET scan lets doctors review metabolic function. Another test called a DaTscan can assess the dopamine transporter. Individuals with MSA do not respond to the drug levodopa that is effective for treating Parkinson's.

WHAT IS THE TREATMENT?

Presently, no treatments can delay the progress of MSA; no cure exists. However, several strategies help people cope with the symptoms. If the person falls faint from hypotension, he or she may be advised to wear compression stockings, drink plenty of water, and avoid heavy meals. Sometimes certain drugs may be prescribed. Bladder control problems can also be treated. The person will need help walking. Physical therapy may help maintain mobility, and reduce muscle spasms from a sedentary life.

For Further Information

Wenning, Gregor K., and Alessandra Fanciulli, eds. *Multiple System Atrophy*. New York: Springer, 2014.

Myasthenia Gravis: Serious Muscle Weakness

- Main symptom is extreme muscle weakness
- Incidence: 3 to 30 cases per million per year
- Can develop at any age; most cases involve women between the ages of 20 to 40, and men between the ages 50 and 60
- Generally considered an autoimmune disease

Gertrude, 93, began to have unusual symptoms at age 60. Her muscles became tired and weak, and she noticed that her eyes began to "sink back in her head." Old age, she thought. It was not until she had a crisis in which she could not breathe that the doctors said to her, "You have myasthenia gravis."

WHAT IS MYASTHENIA GRAVIS?

Myasthenia gravis (MG) is a chronic neuromuscular condition in which the voluntary or skeletal muscles become very weak. The person becomes tired easily. At first, it is similar to other conditions, and usually is not detected early. The condition is thought to be an autoimmune condition with some genetic possibilities, because it tends to run in families. The gene has not been located.

The name comes from both Greek and Latin. The word "myasthenia" is from two Greek roots: *myo*, meaning "muscle," and *asthenia*, meaning "weakness." *Gravis* is a Latin word meaning "severe" or "serious."

When the body is functioning normally, the nerves send messages to the muscles to work and function. The messages are carried by impulses that travel down the nerve and at the nerve endings release a neurotransmitter called acetylcholine. This important neurotransmitter binds to the receptors, activating a muscle contraction. MG occurs when this process breaks down. The transmission of nerve impulses to muscles is interrupted at the place where the nerves and muscles join. The causes are antibodies that block and destroy the receptors for acetylcholine. The antibodies are produced by one's own immune system; hence, the condition is called an autoimmune disease.

WHAT ARE THE SIGNS AND SYMPTOMS?

One of the first symptoms of MG happens in the jaws. When the person is chewing, he or she may note that the jaw muscles are very tired and seem to be weak. Then if the person rests from eating or chewing, the muscles gain strength again. Another beginning symptom occurs in the voluntary muscles that control eyes and eyelids. The person may note that his eyelids are beginning to droop, or that her vision is blurred. Other facial muscles may appear weak, or swallowing may become difficult.

The disease may vary in severity. The symptoms wax and wane. The individual then thinks it was just something temporary, and then suddenly it appears again. These periods are called remission and exacerbation. It may begin in the facial groups, but then develop into a more generalized condition within one to two years. Other muscle groups are affected. The person becomes unstable and develops a waddling gait, has shortness of breath and difficulty breathing, has impaired speech, and weakness in arms, hands, fingers, and neck. If the muscles for breathing are affected, the person may have a myasthenia crisis, which is life-threatening.

HOW IS IT DIAGNOSED?

The diagnosis can be quite difficult, because the symptoms are similar to other autoimmune disorders. Diagnosis is often missed or delayed, because the symptoms may become better, but then worsen. The history of the person is taken, and the physician looks for weakness in the eye muscles. A neurological examination is given. If the condition is suspected, several tests may be given. A blood test can determine the existence of antibodies against the acetylcholine receptor.

Some chemical tests can be used to study muscle weakness. The doctor administers edrophonium chloride, which relieves the muscle weakness. The drug blocks the breakdown and increases the levels of acetylcholine where the nerves and muscles join. The response to the test indicates the presence of MG.

Other tests include electromyography, in which muscles are studied with small pulses of electricity and imaging. Another test applies ice to study sensitivity. A pulmonary function test measures the strength of respiration, which will help avoid a crisis.

WHAT IS THE TREATMENT?

Several medications have been developed that are anticholinesterase agents that improve nerve-muscle transmission and strength. Immunosuppressive drugs, such as prednisone and cyclosporine, may be used to suppress the production of abnormal antibodies.

Surgical removal of the thymus may help some people. The thymus is a gland that lies in the chest area beneath the breastbone. It plays a role in the development of the normal immune system. Some people with MG develop tumors in the thymus gland, called thyomas. Although the relationship between MG and the thymus is not clearly understood, surgical removal may help.

For Further Information

Henderson, Ronald E. *Attacking Myasthenia Gravis*. Montgomery, AL: NewSouth Books, 2013.

Neuroblastoma: Cancer in Very Young Children

- Rare cancer of the adrenal glands that arises before birth
- Incidence of about 650 cases each year in the United States

- Occurs in children younger than two years old
- Comprises about 6–10 percent of all childhood cancers and 15 percent of cancer deaths in children

Kaylee and Kyle were very proud of their wonderful baby girl, Maria. She smiled and was a very happy one-year-old. One day when Kaylee was dressing her, she felt an unusual lump in Maria's abdomen. The doctor said that it might go away, "so let's just watch it for a while." But when another lump developed on her head, they knew that it was serious. Although she was being seen at a prestigious children's hospital in Jacksonville, Florida, the doctors insisted she go to a hospital in New York that specializes in treating a rare type of cancer called neuroblastoma. Neuroblastoma is an important disorder that arises before birth.

WHAT IS NEUROBLASTOMA?

Neuroblastoma (NB) is a rare type of cancer that is found in infants and young children under age two. The cancer cells form in the nerve tissue of the adrenal gland, which sit on top of the kidneys, or in the nerve tissue of the neck, chest, and spinal cord. The word "neuroblastoma" comes from three Greek roots: *neuro* meaning "nerve," *blaston* meaning "germ cell," and *oma,* meaning "tumor of." A neuroblast is an embryonic germ cell from which the nerves develop. Although the symptoms may not show up until a year or so later, it usually has developed before the child is born.

In 1864, the famous German physician and researcher Rudolf Virchow (1821–1902) was the first to describe an abdominal tumor. He called it a glioma, a tumor of the glia or tissue that surrounds the nerves. Another German doctor, Felix March-and (1846–1928), specialized in the tumors of the adrenal glands, and found how these tumors were related to the sympathetic nervous system, which controls all the involuntary functions of the body. In 1901, William Pepper (1843–1898), an American physician, described the four stages of this cancer, and in 1910, James Homer Wright (1869–1928), an early and influential American pathologist, found that the tumor originated from primitive nerve cells and gave them the name "neuroblastoma." He was also responsible for finding in bone marrow special cells that looked like little rosettes; these structures are now called Homer–Wright pseudorosettes.

Because of the difficulty in understanding the exact processes of what happens as the embryo develops, the actual cause is not well understood. Most of the cases are sporadic and occur while the embryo is developing. A few genetic possibilities are seen in about 1–2 percent of cases, where there is a family link. Onset possibly occurs soon after conception, and may be influenced by the maternal use of certain chemicals, smoking, and alcohol. One study has linked the mother's use of hair dye with the development of NB in the fetus. All these are still inconclusive.

WHAT ARE THE SIGNS AND SYMPTOMS?

The symptoms may begin with a swollen-looking abdominal area. A caregiver notes a painless, bluish lump in the abdomen or possibly the neck or chest. The previously normal-looking child may develop dark circles around the eyes, and the eyes may bulge. The child may appear lethargic, weak, or unable to move parts of the body and may experience pain in the bones. Other symptoms are less common: fever, shortness of breath, easy bruising, high blood pressure, diarrhea, jerky muscles, uncontrolled eye movements, and swelling of the legs, ankles, or scrotum.

Neuroblastomas can develop anywhere along the chain of the sympathetic nervous system from the head to the pelvis. The NB can spread to other parts of the body before the first symptoms occur, and before the parents are aware of the problem. In fact, 50–60 percent of cases do metastasize to other parts of the body.

HOW IS IT DIAGNOSED?

The first doctor's exam will involve checking general health, and for signs of the disease. Chemistry studies of urine and blood will test for higher than normal amount of the hormones dopamine and norepinephrine. Studies of a sample of the bone marrow will indicate presence of cancer cells and changes in chromosomes. In addition, an X-ray, CT scan, and ultrasound tests will be given.

In 1997, researchers divided the cancer into four stages:

Stage 1—The cancer is confined to the place of origin and has not spread.

Stage 2—This stage is divided into two types. One type indicates a tumor in only one area and all the visible signs are surgically removed. In the second type, all visible signs of the tumor have been removed, but cancer cells are found in the lymph node near the tumor.

Stage 3—One of the following is true: tumor cannot be completely removed and has spread from one side of the body to another, or may be in the lymph nodes; the tumor is in only one area, but has spread to the lymph nodes on the other side of the body; tumor is in the middle of the body and has spread to both sides of the body; growth cannot be removed.

Stage 4—This stage is divided into stage 4 and 4S. In stage 4, the tumor has spread to distant lymph nodes and to other parts of the body. In stage 4S, the child is younger than a year old; cancer has spread to skin, liver, and bone marrow, but not into bone itself. The primary tumor in only one area, and all the tumors in that location, can be completely removed during surgery, and/or cancer cells may be found in the lymph nodes near the primary tumor.

WHAT IS THE TREATMENT?

For treatment, the types of cancer are divided into 3 risk groups:

Low risk—Those that have an excellent chance of being cured.

Intermediate risk—Those that have a good chance of being healed.

High risk—Those that may be difficult to cure.

A large team of doctors led by a pediatric oncologist will look at the treatment possibilities. According to the results of a battery of tests, the doctors can decide upon the following strategies:

- **Surgery.** This is the usual treatment, depending on where the tumor is and whether or not it has spread.
- **Radiation therapy.** Using high energy X-rays and other types of radiation may kill the cancer cells.
- **Chemotherapy.** The way that chemotherapy is given depends upon the kinds and stage of cancer.
- **Watchful waiting.** No treatment is given until symptoms have changed.
- **Monoclonal antibody therapy.** Antibodies are made in the laboratory and may attach to cancer cells.
- **High-dose chemotherapy and radiation therapy with stem cell transplant.** Stem cells are taken from the person's own body, and these cells migrate to the bone marrow to enable it to make blood cells.
- **Other drug therapy** such as 13-*cis* retinoid acid.

For Further Information

Ormsby, Rachel A. *Learning to Dance in the Rain: A Parent's Guide to Neuroblastoma Diagnosis, Treatment and Beyond.* Printed by CreateSpace, 2013.

Oral Allergy Syndrome: Mixed Messages from the Immune System

- Type of allergy characterized by reactions in the mouth when eating certain foods that may cross-interact with certain pollens
- Most common food-related allergy in adults

- Over one-third of people who have pollen allergies also have this response to certain fruits, vegetables, and some tree nuts
- Reactions may be mild or life-threatening

A person bites into a juicy peach or orange, and several minutes later, her mouth feels itchy and irritated. She is aware that she has a pollen allergy that seems to happen every spring when trees, grasses, and flowers are blooming. But what is happening in the mouth is the result of the immune system sending mixed messages that are the result of oral allergy syndrome.

According to the American College of Allergy, Asthma, and Immunology, about one-third of those with pollen allergies have oral allergy syndrome. This is a real allergy, and one that people know little about.

WHAT IS ORAL ALLERGY SYNDROME?

Oral allergy syndrome (OAS) is a type of allergy reflected by a cluster of reactions in the mouth after eating certain foods that have a similar chemical structure to certain pollens. OAS usually starts in older children and teens, but then continues into adulthood as individuals are exposed to certain types of foods.

The immune system produces antibodies that fight off certain infections by binding to those foreign invaders. One type of antibody is immunoglobulin-E or IgE. Allergies occur when a person's system has been sensitized by an allergen, and antibodies are produced that will come to the body's defense when they encounter the allergen. However, sometimes the reaction will not be helpful, and the person develops an allergy. OAS is an actual allergy, and is called Type 1 or Ig-E-mediated immune response. In OAS, the immune function produces antibodies that bind both to pollen proteins and foods that may have a similar chemical structure. The allergy is not to the food but to the cross-reactivity between remnants of tree of weed pollens that certain fruits and vegetables still have. The immune system produces these Ig-E antibodies against pollen, but they then cross-react with the chemicals found in plants that may be botanically related.

People with OAS can have one or more of the following fruit-pollen associations:

- Ragweed combined with melons, banana, cucumber, sunflower seeds, dandelions, zucchini, and the health foods chamomile tea and Echinacea
- Grass pollen combined with figs, peaches, melons, tomatoes, oranges
- Birch pollen with apples, kiwi, pears, peaches, plums, coriander, fennel, celery, cherries, carrots, hazelnuts, and almonds
- Mugwort (a weed) combined with carrots, celery, coriander, fennel, parsley, peppers, and sunflower

- Possible cross-reactions to any of the above, including berries such as strawberries, blueberries, and raspberries, citrus fruit, mango, figs, peanuts, pineapple, pomegranates, and watermelon

WHAT ARE THE SIGNS AND SYMPTOMS?

A number of allergic reactions may occur, ranging from simple itching that lasts only a few minutes to very serious anaphylactic shock. A person with the syndrome will experience itching, burning, or tingling in areas where the fresh fruit, vegetable, or nut has touched. The person may also have slight swelling and bumpiness of the lips, mouth, ear canal, tongue, and throat. The symptoms usually begin within a few minutes after eating the food, but they may lessen when the food is swallowed. In addition, a person may get some of the symptoms when merely touching or peeling the fruits or vegetables.

Some studies have shown that up to 9 percent of people who have allergies to pollen may have more serious symptoms. If gastric juices do not destroy the food allergen, the person may experience vomiting, diarrhea, cramps, or other gastrointestinal problems. However, about 2 percent may experience anaphylaxis and fall into wheezing, vomiting, hives, and low blood pressure. This is when the person must seek medical help immediately.

HOW IS IT DIAGNOSED?

The person may already know that he has allergies, such as lactose intolerance or other problems that involve metabolizing chemicals. If the person suspects that she has an allergy, she should go to an allergy specialist. The doctor performs a skin prick test, in which the arm or back is scored with a grid. A small amount of different kinds of allergens is then scratched into the area. If a reaction occurs in any of the areas, the person is allergic to that substance.

WHAT IS THE TREATMENT?

The symptoms may vary with the pollen season and may wax and wane. Avoiding the suspect fruits and vegetables is essential. Usually the fruits and vegetables are tolerated if cooked. A few studies have shown that allergy shots targeting the cross-reacting pollens can eliminate the symptoms.

For Further Information

Konstantinou, G. N., and C. E. H. Grattan. July 2008. "Food Contact Hypersensitivity Syndrome: The Mucosal Contact Urticaria Paradigm." *Clinical & Experimental Dermatology* 33 (4): 383–389.

Paresthesia: That Tingling Feeling

- Unusual sensation of tingling or numbness in limbs
- Arises from nerve compression
- Two kinds: transient and chronic
- Treatment depends on cause

Almost everyone has had the mysterious feeling of "my hand has gone to sleep" or "I must stand up because my foot is tingling." It may arise from sleeping with an arm under the body or sitting too long with legs crossed. Whatever the circumstance, the person is miserable for the moments until he or she gets the relief, which is usually not long. That feeling of the foot falling asleep is called paresthesia.

WHAT IS PARESTHESIA?

Paresthesia is a condition in which there is a sensation of tingling, burning, or numbness on the person's skin, with no apparent cause. Usually it occurs in the extremities, especially in the hands, fingers, feet, or toes. It can also occur in other parts of the body, with the feeling that the skin is crawling.

The word "paresthesia" comes from two Greek words *para,* meaning "beside" and *aesthesia,* meaning "feeling." The same root word *esthesia* is also found in the common word anesthesia, which means "without feeling."

Basically, there are two kinds of paresthesia: transient and chronic.

Transient paresthesia. This type is the uncomfortable "pins and needles" feeling that comes from cutting off the blood supply to the nerves. The most common is resting or leaning on a body part that will put stress on the nerves in a certain area. For example, sleeping with an arm under the body may cut off the supply of nerves to the hands and fingers. Riding in a car or plane for a long period of time may put pressure on the circulatory system that nourishes the nerves to the feet and toes. Usually, movement of the limbs will soon restore the normal circulation.

Two other causes of transient paresthesia are hyperventilating and panic attacks. These may last a little longer but usually subside when the condition is arrested.

Chronic or intermittent paresthesia. This type may result from a condition that causes poor circulation. There is a long list of things that may cause a chronic sensation of numbness or tingling. The tingling arises from real nerve damage from a neurological disease or traumatic injury. Following are the types of conditions that may cause chronic paresthesia:

- **Disorders affecting the central nervous system.** Included here are strokes, mini-strokes (called transient ischemic attacks or TIAs), multiple sclerosis, peripheral neuropathy, sciatica, and encephalitis. A whiplash injury from an accident may put pressure on nerves.

- **Tumors.** The growths press against the brain or spinal cord
- **Poor circulation in the limbs** caused by atherosclerosis (buildup of plaques in arteries)
- **Nerve entrapment syndrome**, such as carpal tunnel syndrome
- **Metabolic disorders,** such as diabetes or hypothyroidism
- **Frostbite**
- **Other conditions**, such as herniated disk, Lyme disease, and vitamin B_{12} and B_5 deficiencies

WHAT ARE THE SIGNS AND SYMPTOMS?

The symptoms of paresthesia can be described in many ways. The person may experience tingling, numbness, pins and needles, itching, or burning. Any unusual skin sensation is important in helping the physician make a diagnosis.

HOW IS IT DIAGNOSED?

The simple transient paresthesia is easy to diagnose, because the person experiences tingling and can talk about it. However, the more persistent type may be indicative of some more serious conditions, which need to be investigated.

WHAT IS THE TREATMENT?

The treatment for transient paresthesia is usually simple and easy to do: uncross the legs and rotate the foot or move and shake the hand. No medical assistance is needed here. Although paresthesia itself is rarely life-threatening, it can be the result of a serious condition such as stroke. If a person has such sensations combined with loss of bladder control, or weakness on a part of the body, he or she should get immediate medical attention.

For Further Information

"NINDS Paresthesia Information Page." National Institute of Neurological Disorder and Stroke. http://www.ninds.nih.gov/disorders/paresthesia/paresthesia.htm.

Pickwickian Syndrome: Obese and Unable to Breathe

- Also known as obesity hypoventilation syndrome (OHS)
- Related to morbid obesity

- Obese people breathe poorly and do not get enough oxygen
- Person is sleepy and drowsy all the time, except when eating

Fat Joe had a red, red face. He was traveling in a coach with Mr. Pickwick when soldiers started firing mortars at them, but Joe slept through the entire attack. Joe did wake up when it was time to eat, and gulped down a fat capon and veal patties. Then he went back to sleep and snored loudly.

If you're familiar with Charles Dickens's novel *The Posthumous Papers of the Pickwick Club,* you'll recognize Joe, the portly character with the incredible ability to fall asleep anytime, anywhere . . . unless he's eating. In 1956, Dr. C. S. Burwell (1893–1964), a Harvard professor, in a medical journal applied the term Pickwickian syndrome to one of his patients, a business executive who stood five-feet-five inches, weighed over two-hundred-sixty pounds and had symptoms similar to Joe's. In the 1960s, various other discoveries described these conditions as sleep apnea and sleep hypoventilation.

Statistics from the Centers for Disease Control and Prevention show that sixty million Americans are extremely obese. So it's no surprise that Pickwickian syndrome is on the rise.

WHAT IS PICKWICKIAN SYNDROME?

Pickwickian syndrome, medically called obesity hypoventilation syndrome (OHS), is a disorder in which obese people breathe so poorly that they cannot get enough oxygen, which in turn leads to higher carbon dioxide levels in the blood. The disease strains the heart and can cause heart failure. The term "hypoventilation" comes from the Greek roots *hypo* meaning "under" and *ventilatos* meaning "wind."

The exact cause of this syndrome is really not known. It does have to be connected in some way to morbid obesity. The symptoms are believed to be caused by some misconnection in the brain that controls breathing. That combined with the excessive weight against the chest wall interrupts normal breathing. The pressure against the chest wall makes it difficult for the person to breathe in and expand the lungs to take in oxygen. Therefore, the proper oxygen-carbon dioxide exchange cannot take place. Oxygen does not make it into the bloodstream and the waste carbon dioxide is not expelled properly. Thus, carbon dioxide is kept in the blood, causing a condition known as respiratory acidosis.

People with Pickwickian syndrome may also have a form of sleep apnea or obstructive sleep disorder. They wake up from sleep in brief periods gasping for air. Because of the ensuing oxygen shortage, the brain tells the person to wake up and breathe. The cycle is repeated hundreds of times a night. All this puts a strain on the heart. A recent study in the *New England Journal of Medicine* revealed obstructive sleep apnea elevates the risk of stroke and death, and patients may be prone to falling asleep while driving, increasing the chance of an accident.

WHAT ARE THE SIGNS AND SYMPTOMS?

Although the exact cause of the syndrome is not known, the person's obesity obviously has some affect. Excessive weight pushes against the chest, making it hard for the person to breathe. The body cells are getting too little oxygen, and thus the carbon dioxide level increases. Obesity is the primary risk factor.

Following are the main symptoms:

- The person is sleepy and very drowsy during the day.
- He is tired after exerting little or no effort.
- She has shortness of breath and breathes heavily.
- He complains of headaches, which occur when the brain does not get enough oxygen.
- She is depressed.
- His lips, fingers, toes, and skin take on a bluish color, a condition called cyanosis.
- Her face has a red color.
- There are signs of the failure of the right side of the heart, a condition called cor pulmonale. This may result in swollen feet or legs.

HOW IS IT DIAGNOSED?

Pickwickian syndrome is diagnosed by a combination of the following: obesity (body mass index 30 kg/m 2), hypoxia or falling oxygen levels in the blood during sleep, and hypercapnia or increased levels of carbon dioxide in the blood during the day. Tests for diagnosis include taking arterial blood gas, chest X-ray or CT scan to rule out other causes, lung function tests, and a sleep study. Doctors can tell the difference between just normal obstructive sleep apnea and Pickwickian syndrome, because these patients with OHS have high carbon dioxide levels in the blood when awake.

WHAT IS THE TREATMENT?

To treat the symptoms, a noninvasive ventilation machine called a continuous positive airway pressure or CPAP may be used. Oxygen may also be administered. However, these treatments may be only temporary, and the person will eventually need to consider weight loss.

For Further Information

Olson A. L., and C. Zwillich. 2005. "The Obesity Hypoventilation Syndrome." *American Journal of Medicine* 118 (9): 948–56.

Raynaud's Phenomenon: Reaction to the Cold

- Affects blood vessels in fingers and toes in response to cold
- Prevalence: About 5 percent of the U.S. population
- Primary cause is unknown
- Secondary cause related to a number of other diseases

Raynaud's syndrome is a rare disorder that affects the blood vessels in the fingers and toes, in response to cold. The skin in the affected area turns white, then blue. The cause of the primary type is unknown; a secondary type may be related to a number of diseases.

WHAT IS RAYNAUD'S PHENOMENON?

Raynaud's (pronounced ray-NOZ) phenomenon is a condition that occurs when the arteries narrow reducing the flow of blood to the extremities in response to cold. The term "vasospasm" is used to describe what happens. For some unknown reason, the blood vessels narrow and constrict. It is like having a constricting rubber band cut off the circulation to the areas. When the contracting band is taken off, the finger will be numb, throb, and turn red. This response is similar to what happens in Raynaud's. Although other areas such as the nose, ears, lips, tongue, and nipples can be affected, most of the cases affect the fingers with about 40 percent affecting the toes.

Some confusion may exist about the names: phenomenon, disease, or syndrome. Actually, there are two types of Raynaud's phenomenon. By itself, "Raynaud's phenomenon" simply refers to the reduced blood flow and response to cold. When Raynaud's is linked with the word disease, it is known as primary Raynaud's, the cause of which is unknown. When linked with syndrome, it is known as secondary Raynaud's, and is related to a number of other diseases. Both types respond to cold, and even a slight change in temperature or even something as simple as getting food from a freezer may trigger it. The temperature that appears to be the point of attack is below 60°F.

Maurice Raynaud (1834–1881) was a French physician who worked in several hospitals in Paris. He marveled that humans really are tropical animals, and they can respond to cold by putting on clothes. However, some of his patients had difficulty with cold weather. In 1862, Raynaud described the symptoms of a clinical syndrome in which some people respond abnormally to cold. He wrote about how the digits become white then blue or cyanotic, then turn red when the circulation returns. For his work in this area, the condition was named after him.

Following are the two types of Raynaud's phenomenon and their causes:

- **Primary or Raynaud's disease.** Sometimes this is referred to as being "allergic to the cold." This type is idiopathic, which means the conditions appear to occur by themselves with no distinct cause. They do not appear with other diseases. Women appear to have the condition more frequently than men, and the first episodes probably occurred when they were teenagers or young adults. Some scientists think that there is a hereditary component, but they have never found a gene or combination of genes that are responsible. Others think hormones may play a role. Certain lifestyle choices may increase the attacks. Habits such as smoking and consuming a lot of caffeine may increase the intensity of the attacks.
- **Secondary or Raynaud's syndrome.** This syndrome may be more difficult to manage. Knowing the underlying disease is extremely important. There are a number of diseases that are associated with Raynaud's syndrome. Following are groups of diseases and conditions that may be connected:
  1. Connective tissues disorders, such as scleroderma, lupus, rheumatoid arthritis, Sjögren's syndrome, or Ehlers-Danlos syndrome
  2. Eating disorders such as anorexia nervosa
  3. Certain obstructive disorders such as atherosclerosis
  4. Drugs such as beta-blockers, drugs for chemotherapy, stimulant medications for such conditions such as ADHD, and certain vaccines
  5. Certain jobs that have lots of vibration, such as a power drill operator, or exposure to cold such as in a meat packing plant
  6. And a long list of others that include auto accidents, Lyme disease, and multiple sclerosis

WHAT ARE THE SIGNS AND SYMPTOMS?

Classic Raynaud's goes through all three color changes: white, blue, and then red when recovering. In addition, there is pain and numbness. Milder cases can exist where all these colors do not occur; it depends on the degree of the vasoconstriction. Someone with either type of Raynaud's should be extremely cautious when going to an extremely cold climate. Those who have severe Raynaud's can develop skin sores or gangrene if the attacks are repeated, and it can be fatal. However, most people do not have long-term disability or damage.

HOW IS IT DIAGNOSED?

Diagnosing the disorder can be difficult. Physicians will have to consider a long list of secondary diseases. A variety of tests are now given; however, none are completely satisfactory.

WHAT IS THE TREATMENT?

Some drugs that work to keep the blood vessels open have been found to be effective in some cases. However, researchers are looking for better ways to diagnose and treat the condition. A 2009 article in *Plastic and Reconstructive Surgery* described good results using Botox injections with severe Raynaud's.

For Further Information

Wigley, Fredrick M., Ariane L. Herrick, and Nicholas A. Flavahan, eds. *Raynaud's Phenomenon: A Guide to Pathogenesis and Treatment*. New York: Springer, 2014.

Savants: People Who Can Do Extraordinary Feats

- Also known as autistic savants and idiot savants (a term no longer used)
- People who possess capacities far in excess of what would be normal
- Rare among those with autism
- Savant syndromes may also occur in people with other developmental disabilities

In the movie *Rain Man,* Dustin Hoffman plays the part of Raymond Babbitt, a man with autism who has unusual skills and a tremendous memory. He is able to quote statistics, recite pages of the telephone book, and count cards in Las Vegas. The film brought the term "autistic savant" into the minds of the public.

WHAT IS A SAVANT?

A savant is a person who demonstrates extraordinary mental abilities beyond those expected of a normal person. The syndrome is rare and found in some—but not all—people who have autistic spectrum disorder, other mental disabilities, or injuries to the nervous system.

Individuals who can do extraordinary feats have always fascinated others. John Langdon Down (1828–1896), a Cornish physician, was one of the first to study children born with birth defects. He attempted to classify these individuals according to ethnicity and wrote a paper in 1866, "Observations on the Ethnic Classification of Idiots." He classified people with Mongoloid characteristics as "the Mongolian type of idiot." The name Down syndrome was named for him, and at that time, people with the syndrome were referred to as mongoloids. In 1887 he first described and used the term "idiot savant." When using these words, he was not demeaning the person but simply trying to classify the individual. He stated that although these children were "feeble-minded," they displayed extraordinary skills and special faculties. He then described a number of cases of children who had numerical and musical skills. One of his patients had memorized large portions of Gibbon's *The Decline and Fall of the Roman Empire* and could quote them verbatim.

Today the term "idiot savant" is harsh and unacceptable. Some individuals have referred to the condition as "autistic savant," however, not all savants are autistic. Some have other developmental disorders or brain damage. The preferred term now is just "savant." The term is not listed in *The Diagnostic and Statistical Manual of Mental Disorders*, fifth edition (*DSM-5*) or in the European International Classification of Diseases, 10th revision (ICD-10).

There is no widely accepted explanation for savants. Some people believe that the individual with autism has an uncanny ability to focus and systematize. CT (computed tomography) and MRI (magnetic resonance imaging) scans only show that there is a deficit in one area of the brain, but the scans do not really explain it. The neurological explanation is that there is damage to the left-anterior temporal lobe, which is key to certain memory and sensory input. Scientists have created special transgenic mice by manipulating this area of the brain; these mice display similar mouse savant syndromes.

WHAT ARE THE SIGNS AND SYMPTOMS?

Savantism always involves some unusual feat, and falls within the categories of exceptional mathematical calculations, memory feats, artistic abilities, or musical ability. For example, the person may be asked to tell what day of the week a specific date fell upon. Others may be able to mentally calculate large numbers or square roots.

HOW IS IT DIAGNOSED?

Diagnosis is fairly obvious. The person will be able to do feats that others cannot, and not be able to do other feats that most people can.

WHAT IS THE TREATMENT?

Actually the best treatment may be no treatment. When many of these individuals are studied with the effort to harness the talent in some way, the abilities tend to disappear.

FIVE FASCINATING SAVANTS

1. **Kim Peek.** Most of us have not heard this name, but the life of this person is the one that the movie *Rain Man* was based on. Kim was brain damaged at birth, and his developmental disorders were so serious that the doctor recommended placing him in a home and forgetting about him. His family did not do this. He has read over 12,000 books and can read two pages at once—with one eye on one page and the other on the other page. He remembers details in 15 fields from history to sports, and remembers every piece of music he has ever heard. Still Kim cannot button his shirt and has difficulty walking.

2. **Leslie Lemke.** Leslie was severely brain damaged at birth, and his eyes had to be removed. His mother did not want him, and so he was adopted by a 52-year-old nurse. He did not walk until he was 12. When he was 16, his adoptive mother heard Tchaikovsky's Piano Concerto No. 1 being played in their home one night. Leslie had heard the piece once on television and was able to play it flawlessly on the piano. He began to play all kinds of music, from classical to ragtime. He gave concerts around the world.

3. **Gottfried Mind.** This young boy was one of the earliest savants in history. He went to art school in 1776, where the teacher said his talent was very weak. One day a teacher drew a cat, and Gottfried exclaimed that that was not a real cat. He proceeded to draw a cat that was extremely lifelike. He became known as "the Cat Raphael."

4. **Daniel Tammet.** This boy looked very normal, but was classified as a high functioning autistic savant with exceptional mathematical and language abilities. He was first recognized when he recited from memory the mathematical term pi to 22.514 decimal places. He has a special form of synthesia in which he sees numbers, colors, shapes, and textures. He speaks 11 languages, including Icelandic. He may be different from other savants, in that he can explain the actual methods and procedures of how he works.

5. **Orlando Serrell.** When Orlando was 10, he was hit on the left side of the head by a baseball and suffered brain damage. After he recovered, he found he could do unusual calculations in his head. He could perform complex calendar calculations, and remember the weather of every day, beginning with that day in 1979 when he was hit by the baseball.

For Further Information

Treffert, Darold A. *Extraordinary People: Understanding Savant Syndrome.* Printed by Back-inprint.com, 2006.

Sjögren Syndrome: How Dry I Am

- An autoimmune disease that has several symptoms, including dryness in eyes, mouth, and other body parts
- Affects one in 70 Americans; 9 out of 10 are women
- Third most common autoimmune disease after lupus and multiple sclerosis
- Treatment is only symptomatic

Venus Williams is an American professional tennis player who is a former World Number 1. She was the first African American woman to accomplish this feat, and is credited with bringing the game into a new era of power and athleticism. Williams began to get tired easily, and felt that her fatigue was affecting her performance. In 2011, she was diagnosed with Sjögren syndrome, forcing her to withdraw from the U.S. Open before her second-round match. After the diagnosis, she adopted a vegan diet and reduced her intake of calories and sugar. She also now is engaged in her other passion, interior design. Williams has worked hard to cope with this disorder and is still participating in tennis competition.

WHAT IS SJÖGREN SYNDROME?

Sjögren syndrome (SS) is an autoimmune disorder that mostly affects people over the age of 40, but can be found at any age. For the individual with SS, life is a series of physical complaints that makes daily life painful and difficult. An autoimmune disorder occurs when the body's white blood cells destroy certain glands or cells. SS targets those glands that produce saliva and tears. This leads to dry mouth and dry eyes, and eventually damages the glands. The condition can be either primary, occurring by itself, or secondary, occurring in conjunction with another autoimmune disorder.

In 1930 a Swedish eye doctor Henrik Sjögren (1899–1986) observed a person who had low secretion from the tear and salivary glands. In a 1933 doctoral thesis studying 19 females, he introduced the term keratoconjunctivitis sicca, which means dry eye. Later, in 1950, he expanded the study to 80 women with dry eye, 50 of whom had arthritis. His name became associated with the syndrome.

The actual cause of the syndrome is unknown. However, scientists consider several things. In families that have SS, there is a prevalence of genetic disorders. Mutations occur in the human leukocyte antigen (HLA) region of the genome. However, studies show that the inheritance pattern is not simple like in cystic fibrosis; the relationship is much more complex, indicating a number of factors or other environmental factors. Environmental factors may include certain viruses, such as the Epstein-Barr virus (EBV), hepatitis C, or human T-cell leukemia. Hormones factors may also be involved. Because so many of the patients are women, estrogen or other sex hormones may be involved.

WHAT ARE THE SIGNS AND SYMPTOMS?

The main symptoms include generalized dryness or sicca syndrome. *Sicca* is the Latin word for dry. Dry eye or keratoconjunctivitis sicca usually is one of the first specific complaints. The person experiences frequent eye infections, has difficulty focusing, and eye pain. The eyes may have a gritty sensation, as if there is a foreign body in the eye. The eyes may be very red and itchy, with an added sensitivity to light that makes watching television very difficult. In addition, the individual may have dry mouth, which can include complications of dental decay, oral pain, and infection. The lack of saliva makes it difficult to chew, swallow, and speak. Patients may find they are sipping water continuously. The syndrome may also include dry skin, nose, and vagina, and eventually affect other organs, such as the kidneys, blood vessels, lungs, liver, pancreas, peripheral nervous system, and brain.

Other symptoms may be more generalized and also can be symptomatic of other diseases. These include fatigue, muscle and joint paint, acid reflux (GERD), difficulty swallowing, sleep disturbance, forgetfulness and other cognitive difficulties, and numbness in the extremities.

HOW IS IT DIAGNOSED?

Due to the wide-ranging set of symptoms, the period of time between the onset of the disease and diagnosis can be as long as six and a half years. Because of the similarity to other conditions, the diagnosis is considered difficult. Blood tests can determine high levels of antibodies that are indicative of the condition. Other tests can measure the function of the lacrimal glands, the production of tears, and the salivary glands.

WHAT IS THE TREATMENT?

Currently, there is no cure nor a specific treatment for permanent recovery. Treatment is symptomatic and supportive. For example, dry eye can be treated with artificial tears. Cyclosporine (Restasis) is effective in suppressing inflammation and chronic dry eye. Also, prescription drugs such as cevimeline (Evoxac) can help produce saliva in the mouth and intestine. Anti-inflammatory drugs may be used to treat muscle and skeletal symptoms. Dental care is extremely important, because lack of saliva can cause tooth decay and other problems.

For Further Information
Wallace, Daniel J., ed. *The Sjögren's Book*. New York: Oxford University Press, 2013.

Synesthesia: Mixing the Senses

- A neurological condition in which a person experiences "crossed" responses to stimuli
- Prevalence may be as high as 1 in 300 to as low as 1 in 2,000
- Many synesthetes consider their condition a gift
- Has been studied extensively, but underlying cause is still not fully understood

When Patty was a child, she began to realize that some of her senses were different from that of other people. She explained later that when she tried to make the letter P, she would see the color yellow. When she would draw a line down from the loop to make the letter R, she would see it turn into another color—orange. Patty had an unusual ability to see colors in ways that were related to other senses. She has synesthesia and is called a "synesthete."

WHAT IS SYNESTHESIA?

Synesthesia is a neurological condition that occurs when one sensory stimulus may lead to another other sense. It is sometimes defined as union of the senses. The word comes from the Greek: *syn*, meaning "together," and *aesthesia*, meaning "sensation." It is involuntary and automatic, as one sensory pathway leads to a second sense.

Synesthesia was popular as a subject of scientific investigation during the late 19th and early 20th centuries, but was dropped in the 1950s. It has recently been revived with functional neuroimaging (fMRI) and other brain study initiatives.

The Greeks realized that there were people who said that they could hear color. Later Sir Isaac Newton (1643–1727) proposed that musical tones and colors shared the same frequencies. In 1876, a German Gustav Fechner (1801–1887), known as the father of psychophysics, surveyed 73 people who heard letters that were connected with color. Also, British scientist Francis Galton (1822–1911) wrote extensively on the subject as he explored differential psychology. Abandoned for years, the phenomenon began to be studied again in the 1980s by several researchers. With the rise of the internet, groups such as the American Synesthesia Association have revived interest.

The cause of synesthesia is unknown. Scientists do know that certain regions of the brain are given functions for receiving sight, smell, taste, etc. The areas of the brain somehow cross-activate. There also may be acquired forms caused by head trauma, sensory deprivation, or drug use.

WHAT ARE THE SIGNS AND SYMPTOMS?

Some people who have the condition are often unaware they are different from others. Most people report the experiences as pleasant, although there are a few that may have some behavioral consequences. For example, children with Asperger syndrome often experience one or more forms of synesthesia.

About 60 types have been reported, but scientists have evaluated only a few of these. Because it is such a subjective perception, the reports may vary from person to person. The most common form is called grapheme-color synesthesia. In this form, individual letters of the alphabet and numbers are seen shaded with colors. The most common finding is that the letter A is associated with red.

Other colors may show with different letters of the alphabet. However, not all people see the same color with one specific letter. A second common form is called chromesthesia, in which the person associates sounds with colors. Everyday sounds, such as cars honking or people talking, can trigger the color. Other people associate the color with music. Another form is spatial sequence synesthesia (SSS), in which the person sees the number 1 closer to them in space than the number 2. According to studies, these people are able to recall past events and memories in great detail. This may relate to the person who is an autistic savant, who has unusual abilities.

Some other forms are quite rare, and have not been studied as frequently. A number form is a mental map of numbers that appears when a person thinks of numbers. Francis Galton, the father of differential psychology, saw numbers in form as the digits of a clock's face. In the one of the rarest forms, called auditory- tactile synesthesia, certain sounds evoke sensations in various body parts. When looking at behavioral effects, in a form called misophonia synesthesia, the individual may have bad experiences of anger, flight, hatred, or disgust when triggered by specific sounds. One of the episodes of the television show *Criminal Minds* featured a man who saw red, which stood for evil, when certain persons spoke on the telephone; he decided to exterminate them.

HOW IS IT DIAGNOSED?

The person can describe and attribute unusual senses together. It is not recognized in the fifth edition of the *Diagnostic and Statistical Manual of Mental Disorders* (DSM-5).

WHAT IS THE TREATMENT?

There is no treatment, and none may be needed.

VAN GOGH MAY HAVE BEEN A SYNESTHETE

Vincent van Gogh (1853–1890) was a Dutch painter who produced over 2,100 pieces of art in one decade. He is known for his bright colors. In a letter to his brother in 1881, he mentioned that his paintings were somewhat like the sound of a violin or an organ. Many researchers believe that he had synesthesia and Asperger syndrome, which is often linked to the trait of blended senses. "Photoism" is used to describe the shape that synesthetes see in response to other senses. Two paintings of van Gogh's are the most evident of this happening. *The Starry Night* and *Wheatfield with Crows* show these photisms or swirls. His self-portraits also had some of the same type of brush strokes.

Van Gogh sold only one painting during his life. He died at the age of 37, before he saw any success. His mother threw away crates of his work long before he was hailed as an artistic genius.

For Further Information

Leatherdale, Lyndsay. *Synesthesia. The Fascinating World of Blended Senses. Synesthesia and Types of Synesthesia Explained*. Dublin, Ireland: IMB Publishing, 2013.

Vitiligo: Splotches of White on the Skin

- Also known as leucoderma
- Appears as if someone has thrown white paint on the body part, usually the hands, face, or neck
- Melanin, the pigment that gives color to skin, dies or is unable to function
- Common disorder affecting between 0.5 percent and 1 percent of the population; more noticeable in dark-skinned people

When Michael Jackson, the famous pop singer, died in June 2009, news reports after his autopsy showed that he possibly had a skin condition. He had declared often that he did not bleach his skin to make himself appear white. He might have worn his famous glove because of the presence of a skin condition, known as vitiligo. It is a mysterious condition that may appear in several forms. There is some evidence that it might be inherited, but most researchers classify it as an idiopathic disorder, which might be an autoimmune dysfunction.

WHAT IS VITILIGO?

Vitiligo is a condition in which the person has white splotches on the skin, which someone has described as looking as if white paint had been dribbled over the skin. The loss of skin color is caused by loss of function of the melanocytes. Melanocytes are cells in the basal layer, the deepest layer of the epidermis, the outer layer of the skin. Melanocytes produce the pigment melanin, which determines hair and skin color and also protects people from sunlight. Everyone has the same number of melanocytes but the difference between lighter and darker skin tones is the type, amount, and arrangement of the melanocytes.

People with vitiligo have had difficult times in the past and even in some cultures today. For example, in some areas of India, it is referred to as white leprosy, and is especially feared in dark-skinned people, because of the stark contrast. Certain Hindu beliefs in reincarnation hold that the person sinned in a previous life, and is now being punished. Young unmarried Indian women are especially at risk, because those with vitiligo have a slim chance for an arranged married. If the woman develops the condition after marriage, it is grounds for divorce. However, even some people in Western societies may feel stigmatized and become depressed because of their condition.

The reason that vitiligo is placed in this section is that it is basically considered an autoimmune disorder, in which the body's defense system turns against itself and destroys the melanocytes. About 25 percent of the people with this condition have other autoimmune conditions, such as lupus, rheumatoid arthritis, or psoriasis.

There may be a family history in about 30 percent of patients, and both sexes are equally affected. However, the genes that are related to vitiligo are also those that are seen in autoimmune disorders. There are two main genes:

- *NLRP1* gene. Mutations in this gene are located on the short arm (p) of chromosome 17. The proteins made by this gene are essential to helping the immune system fight inflammation.
- *PTPN22.* Mutations in this gene are located on the short arm (p) of chromosome 1. This gene normally instructs for information that regulates T-cells, part of the immune system.

However, the other 70 percent of cases are idiopathic, and are not traced to a specific cause. It is thought to be a malfunction of the immune system that attacks the melanocytes.

WHAT ARE THE SIGNS AND SYMPTOMS?

The most obvious symptom is depigmentation of patches of skin. The patches may start small and then grow and even change shape. Loss is most noticeable on the face and appears to gather especially around the mouth, eyes, and nostrils. The hands and face are especially vulnerable. However, the patches may appear anywhere on the body, even on the genitals and umbilicus. Some lesions may have a dark outline of hyperpigmentation around the edges.

Most people experience the loss of pigment before they reach the age of 20. And although they may be in good health, they are at risk for developing several autoimmune disorders, such as thyroid issues, vitamin B_{12} deficiency, adrenal problems, hair loss, and problems with the eyes.

Following are the types of vitiligo:

- **Generalized vitiligo.** This most common type has loss of pigment in patches all over the body. It will appear in both the areas that can be seen, such as face and hands, as well as other parts of the body.
- **Segmented vitiligo.** This type has patches on the underside of the body in a segmented fashion.
- **Focal vitiligo.** This type appears only in a specific area. It may be on the face, neck, or trunk. Later in life it may progress to a generalized type.

- **Acrofacial vitiligo.** Pigment is lost on the fingers and face.
- **Trichrome vitiligo.** In this type, there are large patches without color, intermixed with colored skin in between.

HOW IS IT DIAGNOSED?

In addition to the obvious symptoms, diagnosis may also include a skin biopsy and observation with a UVA black light called a Wood's lamp. Skin with vitiligo will glow yellow, green, or blue; those with healthy skin will show nothing.

WHAT IS THE TREATMENT?

The person with vitiligo must constantly take care about going out into the sun. Makeup can cover some of the spots, and bleaching of the skin may be done to create a more uniform color. Physicians may treat with a combination of creams, such as steroid creams, and use of UVB or UVA lamps. In October 1992, the first transplant of melanocytes was performed. At the time, the trial had a 70 percent to 85 percent success rate.

For Further Information

National Institute of Skin Diseases. *VITILIGO: Symptoms, Causes, Diagnosis and Effective Treatments—Official Guide from the National Institute of Skin Diseases.* Washington, DC: National Institutes of Health, 2008.

Helpful Resources for the Study of Unusual Diseases and Disorders

A number of sites are available on the web for additional study. The sites included here are those that are medically sound and are research-based. Also included are a number of books that focus on specific diseases and disorders.

GENERAL RESEARCH

The Family Practice Notebook. http://fpnotebook.com

Medline Plus. http://www.nlm.nih.gov/medlineplus/healthtopics.html (From the National Library of Medicine)

Medscape Reference. http://reference.medscape.com/Medscape

Merck Manual Online. http://merckmanuals.com.home/index.html. Merck also has a hard copy of the manual, published by W.B. Saunders.

Taber's Cyclopedic Medical Dictionary. Clayton Thomas, MD, ed. Philadelphia: F.A. Davis Company, 2001.

WebMD. http://www.webmd.com

UNUSUAL GENETIC DISORDERS

General

Gene Reviews. http://ncbi.nlm.nih.gov/books/NBK1116

Genetic and Rare Diseases Information Center (GARD) http://rarediseases.info.nih.gov /GARD

Kelly, Evelyn B. *Encyclopedia of Human Genetics and Diseases* (two volumes). Santa Barbara, CA: ABC-CLIO, 2013.

Lewis, Ricki. *Human Genetics: Concepts and Applications,* 10th edition. New York: McGraw Hill, 2012.

Marion, Robert. *Genetic Rounds: A Doctor's Encounters in the Field that Revolutionized Medicine.* New York: Kaplan Press, 2009.

Achondroplasia

Nicoletti, B., E. Ascani, V. A. McKusick, and S. C. Dryburgh, eds. *Human Achondroplasia: A Multidisciplinary Approach.* New York: Basic Life Sciences (Springer), 1998.

Amyotrophic Lateral Sclerosis (Lou Gehrig's Disease)

Wakefield, Darcy. *I Remember Running: The Year I Got Everything I Ever Wanted—and ALS.* Boston: DeCapo Press, 1996.

Angelman Syndrome

The Official Parent's Sourcebook on Angelman Syndrome: A Revised and Updated Directory for the Internet Age. Las Vegas, NV: Icon Health Publications, 2005.

Ankylosing Spondylitis

Cousins, Norman. *Anatomy of an Illness: As Perceived by the Patient* (Twentieth Anniversary Edition). New York: WW. Norton, 2005.

Khan, Muhammad Asim, *Ankylosing Spondylitis: The Facts* (The Facts Series). Oxford, UK: Oxford University Press, 2002.

Cri-du-Chat Syndrome

Parker, M. *Cri-Du-Chat Syndrome - A Bibliography and Dictionary for Physicians, Patients.* San Diego, CA: ICON Health Publications, 2007.

Fatal Familial Insomnia

Guilleminault, Christian, *Fatal Familial Insomnia: Inherited Prion Diseases, Sleep, and the Thalamus.* New York: Raven Press, 1994.

Hemochromatosis

Gamson, Cheryl. *The Iron Disorders Institute Guide to Hemochromatosis.* Toronto: Cumberland House, 2009.

Porphyria

Deats-O'Reilly, Diana. *Porphyria: The Unknown Disease.* Grand Forks, ND: Porphyrin Press, 1998.

Prader-Willi Syndrome

Whittington, Joyce, and Tony Holland. *Prader-Willi Syndrome: Development and Manifestation.* New York: Cambridge University Press, 2011.

UNUSUAL MENTAL DISORDERS

General

American Psychiatric Association. *Diagnostic and Statistical Manual of Mental Disorders*, 5th ed. Arlington, VA: American Psychiatric Association, 2013.

National Institute of Mental Health: http://www.nimh.nih.gov.

Noll, Richard. *Bizarre Diseases of the Mind*. New York: Berkley, 1990.

Sacks, Oliver. *Hallucinations*. London: Pan MacMillan UK, 2012.

Alien Hand Syndrome

Bellows, Alan. *Alien Hand Syndrome*. New York: Workman Publishing, 2009.

Capgras Delusion

Vaknin, Sam. *The Capgras Shift*. Rhinebeck, NY: Narcissus Publications, 2011.

Dissociative Identity Disorder

Haddock, Deborah. *The Dissociative Identity Disorder Sourcebook*. New York: McGraw Hill, 2001.

Walker, H. *Breaking Free: My Life with Dissociative Identity Disorder*. New York: Simon and Schuster, 2008.

Erotomania

Orion, Doreen R. *I Know You Really Love Me: A Psychiatrist's Journal of Erotomania, Stalking, and Obsessive Love*. New York: Macmillan, 1997.

Hybristophilia

Parker, R. J. *Serial Killer Groupies*. Toronto: R. J. Parker Publishing, 2014.

Kleptomania

Goldman, Marcus J. *Kleptomania: The Compulsion to Steal—What Can Be Done?* Far Hills, NJ: New Horizon Press, 1997.

Munchausen Syndrome

Feldman, Marc D. *Playing Sick?: Untangling the Web of Munchausen Syndrome, Munchausen by Proxy, Malingering, and Factitious Disorder*. London: Routledge Press, 2004.

Pica

Connor, Jane. *Pica Eating—Overcoming Pica Eating Disorder for Life*. Printed by Amazon Digital Services, 2013.

Stockholm Syndrome

Borst, Kelsi. *Stockholm Syndrome*. Bloomington, IN: AuthorHouse, 2008.

UNUSUAL ENVIRONMENTAL DISEASES AND DISORDERS

General

Norman, Robert. *The Blue Man and Other Stories of the Skin*. Berkeley, CA: University of California Press, 2014.

Nagami, Pamela. *Bitten: True Medical Stories of Bites and Stings*. New York: St. Martin's Griffin, 2004.

Altitude Sickness

Dremousis, Litsa. *Altitude Sickness*. Portland, OR: Instant Future Press, 2013.

Argyria

Hill, John. *Colloidal Silver Medical Uses, Toxicology & Manufacture*. Ranier, WA: Clear Springs Press, 2009.

Histoplasmosis

Daniel, Thomas M., and Gerald L. Baum. *Drama and Discovery: The Story of Histoplasmosis*. Santa Barbara, CA: Praeger, 2002.

Pellagra

Jarrow, Gail. *Red Madness: How a Medical Mystery Changed What We Eat*. Honesville, PA: Calkins Creek, 2014.

Pneumoconiosis

Kee, Kenneth. *A Simple Guide to Pneumoconiosis, Treatment and Related Diseases*. Printed by Amazon Digital Services, 2014.

Stachybotrys

Progovitz, Richard F. *Black Mold: Your Health and Your Home*. Cleveland, NY: Forager Press, 2003.

Thalidomide Embryopathy

Paul, Annie Murphy. *Origins: How the Nine Months Before Birth Shape the Rest of Our Lives*. New York: Free Press, 2011.

Trench Foot

Bull, Stephen. *Trench: A History of Trench Warfare on the Western Front*. Oxford, UK: Osprey Publishing, 2014.

UNUSUAL INFECTIOUS DISEASES

General

Infectious Diseases: MedlinePlus – National Library of Medicine. www.nlm.nih.gov /medlineplus/infectiousdiseases.html.

Moalem, Sharon. *Survival of the Sickest*. New York: Harper Collins, 2007.

Nagami, Pamela. *The Woman with a Worm in her Head and Other True Stories of Infectious Disease*. New York: St. Martin's Press, 2001.

World Health Organization. Infectious diseases.www.who.int.

Cat Scratch Disease

Eldredge, Debra M. *Cat Owner's Home Veterinary Handbook,* 3rd ed. New York: Howell Book House (Wiley), 2007.

Chikungunya

Renn, Liam. *Chikungunya Virus - The New Reality: Your Next Vacation Could Make You Sick for Years*. Printed by Amazon Digital Services, 2015.

Ebola

Preston, Richard. *The Hot Zone*. New York: Anchor Books, 2014.

Enterovirus-D68

Clark, James. *Enterovirus: The Preppers Guide to Surviving Enterovirus*. Printed by Amazon Digital Services, 2015.

Herpes Zoster

Rosebloom, Ashley. *Shingles: Shingles Symptoms, Treatment, Causes and Cures (How to Treat Shingles/Herpes Zoster Virus Book 1)*. Printed by Amazon Digital Services, 2014.

Leprosy

Everest, Frank. *Leprosy: Quick Facts about This Misunderstood Disease*. Published by Skin Diseases, Skin Disorders, and Skin Treatments, 2015.

Necrotizing Fasciitis

Roemmele, Jacqueline A. *Surviving the Flesh-Eating Bacteria: Understanding, Preventing, Treating, and Living with Necrotizing Fasciitis*. New York: Avery, 2000.

Norovirus

Stone, Carolyn. *Norovirus: How to Stay Safe*. New York: Eternal Spring Books, 2014.

UNUSUAL DISEASES AND DISORDERS WITH OTHER OR UNEXPLAINED ORIGINS

General

Asherson, Ronald, ed. *Handbook of Systemic Autoimmune Diseases* (10 volumes). http://www.elsevier.com/wps/find/bookdescription.cws_home/BS_HSAD/description#description.

Prusiner, Stanley B. *Madness and Memory: The Discovery of Prions—A New Biological Principle of Disease*. New Haven, CT: Yale University Press, 2014.

Anti-NMDA-Receptor Encephalitis

Cahalan, Susannah. *Brain on Fire: My Month of Madness*. New York: Free Press, 2012.

Bell's Palsy

Nemcoff, Mamie. *Living with Bell's Palsy*. Reseda, CA: Glenneyre Press, 2011.

Bromhidrosis

Bartone, John C., ed. *Human Sweat and Sweating—Normal and Abnormal Including Hyperhidrosis and Bromhidrosis: Index of New Information and Guide-Book for Reference and Research*. Washington, DC: Abbe Pub Association, 2001.

Guillain-Barre Syndrome

Langton, Brian S. *A First Step—Understanding Guillain-Barre Syndrome*. New York: Trafford Publishing, 2006.

Myasthenia gravis

Henderson, Ronald E. *Attacking Myasthenia Gravis*. Montgomery, AL: NewSouth Books, 2013.

Savants

Treffert, Darold A. *Extraordinary People: Understanding Savant Syndrome*. Published by Backinprint.com, 2006.

Sjögren's Syndrome

Wallace, Daniel J. *The Sjögren's Book*. New York: Oxford Press, 2013.

Synesthesia

Leatherdale, Lyndsay. *Synesthesia. The Fascinating World of Blended Senses. Synesthesia and Types of Synesthesia Explained*. Dublin, Ireland: IMB Publishing, 2013.

Vitiligo

National Institute of Skin Diseases. *VITILIGO: Symptoms, Causes, Diagnosis and Effective Treatments – Official Guide from the National Institute of Skin Diseases.* Washington, DC: National Institutes of Health, 2008.

INDEX

ABOUT THE AUTHOR

Dr. Evelyn Kelly, a resident of Ocala, Florida, is a writer and college professor. With a PhD from the University of Florida, she teaches both graduate and undergraduate classes for Saint Leo University. As a writer, she has published over 400 articles; this book, *The 101 Most Unusual Diseases and Disorders*, is her seventeenth.

Dr. Kelly is a community activist in Marion County political affairs, a participant in musical productions of the Ocala Symphony Orchestra, and a volunteer for special causes. She has traveled to 77 countries on all seven continents. She speaks often to groups about topics concerning health and travel.